Assessment in Adapted Physical Education and Therapeutic Recreation

Assessment in Adapted Physical Education and Therapeutic Recreation

Second Edition

Michael Horvat
University of Georgia

Len Kalakian
Mankato State University

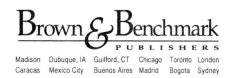

Brown & Benchmark
PUBLISHERS

Madison   Dubuque, IA   Guilford, CT   Chicago   Toronto   London
Caracas   Mexico City   Buenos Aires   Madrid   Bogota   Sydney

Book Team

Executive Managing Editor *Ed Bartell*
Publishing Services Coordinator *Peggy Selle*
Proofreading Coordinator *Carrie Barker*
Visuals/Design Production Manager *Janice Roerig-Blong*
Production Manager *Beth Kundert*
Publishing Services Manager *Sherry Padden*
Visuals/Design Freelance Specialist *Mary L. Christianson*
Marketing Manager *Pam Cooper*
Promotions Manager *Mike Matera*

Basal text: Times Roman
Display type: Helvetica
Typesetting system: Mac/QuarkXPress
Paper Stock: Recycled laser offset
Production Services: Shepherd, Inc.

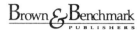

A Times Mirror Higher Education Group Company

President and Chief Executive Officer *Thomas E. Doran*
Vice President/Executive Publisher *Edgar J. Laube*
Vice President/Production and Business Development *Vickie Putman*
Vice President/Sales and Marketing *Bob McLaughlin*

President and Chief Executive Officer *G. Franklin Lewis*
Senior Vice President, Operations *James H. Higby*
Corporate Senior Vice President and President of Manufacturing *Roger Meyer*
Corporate Senior Vice President and Chief Financial Officer *Robert Chesterman*

Consulting Editor *Aileene Lockhart*

Cover design and illustration by Rokusek Design

Copyedited by Shepherd, Inc.

Proofread by Francine Buda Banwarth

This book is dedicated to Drs. Peter Aufsesser, Ron Croce, Len Kalakian, and Glenn Roswal for their loyalty, friendship, and personal and professional support.
                    Michael Horvat

This book is dedicated to Ginny Dahlstrom with love and for reasons that would fill a book; and to Kerby Kalakian, my son, who is also my best friend.
                    Len Kalakian

CONTENTS

8 Assessment of Posture and Gait   129

9 Behavior, Leisure, and Play   148

10   Translating Assessment into Action: A Team Approach   165

Appendix A   Case Studies   186
Index   193

PREFACE

Perhaps the most coveted recognition a textbook author receives from colleagues is peer acceptance of a first edition that warrants undertaking a second edition. In a market as specific as assessment in adapted physical education and therapeutic recreation, peer respect and recognition are the carrots. Only a bad capitalist would ever write for the money.

When Judy Werder and I (LK) undertook the first edition a decade ago, our shared professional goal was to help meet the then long-standing need for clarifying issues surrounding physical and motor assessment of persons with disabilities. In its day, our book made significant strides towards accomplishing our goal. Dr. Werder has since undertaken professional responsibilities that have preempted her collaborating with Dr. Michael Horvat and me in revising this text. Before proceeding any farther, Dr. Horvat and I wish to recognize and thank Dr. Werder for her first edition contributions that remain pillars in the foundation we have endeavored to build on in this second edition.

Pre-service and in-service professionals in therapeutic recreation and adapted physical education engaged in learning or refining assessment skills are the audiences we strive to reach. Professionals in adapted physical education and therapeutic recreation regularly select, administer, and interpret motor tests for numerous related and discrete purposes. Characterized by great variability in purpose, content, difficulty, and format, motor tests (including their selection, administration, and interpretation) generate a vast array of questions in search of answers. Often, simply knowing the questions is the beginning of wisdom. Unfortunately, few textual resources asking questions, endeavoring to answer questions, and clarifying assessment-related issues in adapted physical education and therapeutic recreation are available for use in professional preparation programs. Our continuing goal is to meet a continuing need for clarifying issues surrounding physical and motor assessments of persons who have disabilities. Our specific purpose in revising this text is to provide a significantly updated resource to pre-service and in-service professionals in adapted physical and therapeutic recreation who are developing or fine-tuning their professional motor assessment acumen.

We regard assessment as the cornerstone of any effort to individualize instruction. We present motor assessment as a systematic, multifaceted process of gathering and interpreting information about the student or client. This text endeavors to explain concepts and procedures essential to each therapeutic recreation and adapted physical education specialist's repertoire of professional assessment skills. From our perspective, assessment in adapted physical education and therapeutic recreation, while always challenging, need never be confusing when fundamental principles underlying sound assessment are understood. The therapeutic recreation or adapted physical education specialist who masters concepts presented herein, unlike one who might only administer test items after having only read item administration instructions, will gain credibility as a diagnostician who lights the way with carefully selected tests and thoughtful results interpretation.

The first edition of this text included seven chapters. Chapters appearing in the first edition have been painstakingly updated. In fact, as new information became available, even after the text was in production, that information was interwoven into what the reader will encounter. The second edition, totaling 10 chapters, plus sample cases in Appendix A, additionally or significantly more thoroughly addresses Physical Fitness (Chapter 7), Assessment of Posture and Gait (Chapter 8), Behavior, Leisure, and Play (Chapter 9), and Translating Assessment into Action (Chapter 10).

Development of the second edition of this text represents a continuing effort to provide an authoritative treatise on assessment in adapted physical education and, now, therapeutic recreation. We hope this new edition becomes a well-used, long-lasting resource for college professors, program supervisors, practicing therapeutic recreation specialists and adapted physical educators, and others dedicated to quality physical education and recreation for *all* people.

We wish to thank the reviewers of this text: Dale A. Ulrich, Indiana University; and Bob Rider, Florida State University.

CHAPTER 1

Who Are We Assessing?

Assessment in adapted physical education and therapeutic recreation focuses on identifying activity needs of persons who have disabilities. This needs identification process is essential, because it helps ensure that activity participation is *meaningful*. Two criteria, at minimum, are essential to determine whether participation is, indeed, meaningful. Participation must be (1) safe and (2) successful. Safe and successful participation in mainstream physical education and recreation for persons with disabilities is often (but not always) possible. Among persons with special physical education and recreation needs, a wide range of service options can and should be available. In many instances, pursuant to federal and state mandates, such services *must* be made available. Today, a wide range of modified services provided by adapted physical education (APE) and therapeutic recreation (TR) specialists exists. Options range from the APE or TR specialist serving as consultant for the mainstream service provider to direct service provided wholly by the specialist.

When this text first appeared in 1985, Julien Stein (1979, p. 6) was quoted as follows: "Success and effectiveness in special programs, activities, and efforts should be based upon numbers screened into—not out of regular . . . programs and activities." Stein suggested that potential existed to successfully integrate 90 to 95 percent of persons with disabilities into regular programs. Without question, numbers of persons with disabilities participating in mainstream programs have increased dramatically during the ensuing years. This trend, however, should not be construed as the "swan song" for persons seeking careers in APE or TR. Precisely the opposite is true. Today, more than ever before, persons with special needs are being included in mainstream APE and TR programs. While many, indeed the majority, are being served in the mainstream, a larger than ever number of the total population of persons with disabilities is being served by specialists in APE and TR. Largely because of mandates and an awakening among the general public, persons with disabilities have begun to receive a fair share of program and service opportunities heretofore taken for granted by the general populace. The majority of persons with disabilities today, much to the credit of all concerned, are being included in mainstream programs. What is being experienced among APE and TR specialists is *not* a decline in numbers served. On the contrary, numbers of persons served by APE and TR specialists typically are either stable or increasing. This phenomenon is due largely to dramatic increases in numbers of persons with disabilities in recent years becoming entitled to and seeking special services. Today, APE or TR specialists typically are serving persons with disabilities who are relatively severely or profoundly affected by their disabilities.

Type and extent of disability alone do not determine if a person should be placed in an APE or TR program. Of major significance is the manner in which the individual copes with his or her disability. For example, in myelomeningocele spina bifida, trauma to the spinal cord (an impairment) causes dysfunction (disability) to muscles below the spina bifida site. The disability becomes a *handicap* only when it is identified as a factor that limits choice of lifestyle and pursuit of happiness. All persons with disabilities are not handicapped by their disabilities. Among persons whose disabilities are handicapping, the handicap may present itself only in a few situations or it may be present in most everyday situations. Further, the handicap in question may range from mild to profound. To a great extent, whether a disabling impairment becomes a handicap is determined largely by the person with the disability.

The term *disability*, as used in this text, refers to any condition identified in Public Law 101–476. The term *handicap* is reserved for conditions that result in substantial limitations in one or more significant life activities. Such activities include language (receptive and expressive), self-care, mobility, learning, self-direction, independent living, and economic self-sufficiency.

Role of Public Laws in Determining Who We Assess

Numerous Public Laws have been enacted by the United States Congress, many of which have had as their primary intent the ensurance of full opportunity for persons with disabilities. For assessment in APE and TR purposes, the most significant are addressed below.

Public Law 101–476 (Individuals with Disabilities Education Act [*IDEA*])

IDEA became federal law on October 30, 1990. However, much of what became law with IDEA's passage already had been mandated by Congress with two previously passed federal laws, Public Law 94–142 (*Education of the Handicapped Act of 1975*) and Public Law 99–457 (*Education of the Handicapped Act Amendments of 1986*). Public Law 101–476 combined Public Laws 94–142 and 99–457, and replaced the term "handicap" throughout the new law with the term "disability."

Virtually without question, the most significant legislation today ensuring quality education for young people with disabilities is Public Law 101–476. This law guarantees children with disabilities in the United States, ages 3–21, a free, appropriate education in the least restrictive environment. The law also encourages, though it does not require, states to provide early intervention services for infants and toddlers, ages 0–2, by offering financial incentives to help offset costs of developing and implementing early intervention programs.

Public Law 101–476 identifies specific conditions that, when determined by assessment to adversely affect education, entitle one to federally mandated special education services. All students with disabilities (as defined by Public Law 101–476) who cannot be included meaningfully in the regular curriculum are entitled to individually designed special education and related services. Pursuant to Public Law 101–476, the phrase *children with disabilities* means children (A) with mental retardation, hearing impairments including deafness, speech or language impairments, visual impairments including blindness, serious emotional disturbance, orthopedic impairments, autism, traumatic brain injury, other health impairments or specific learning disabilities; and (B) who, by reason thereof, need special education and related services (PL 101–476, Sec. 1401[a][1]). Disabilities cited above are defined in the *Federal Register* as follows:

I. *Deaf* means a hearing impairment so severe that the child is hindered in processing linguistic information through hearing, with or without amplification, and educational performance is thus adversely affected.

II. *Deaf-blind* means concomitant hearing and visual impairments, the combination of which causes such severe communication and other developmental educational problems that the child cannot be accommodated in special education programs solely for deaf or blind children.

III. *Hard of hearing* means a hearing impairment, whether permanent or not, and is included under the definition of *deaf* in this section.

IV. *Mentally retarded* means significantly subaverage general intellectual functioning that exists concurrently with deficits in adaptive behavior, is manifested in the developmental period, and adversely affects the child's educational performance.

V. *Multihandicapped* means concomitant impairments (e.g., mentally retarded-blind, mentally retarded-orthopedically impaired), the combination of which causes such severe educational problems that the child cannot be accommodated in special education programs designed solely for children with one of the impairments. The term does not include deaf-blind children.

VI. *Orthopedically impaired* means a severe orthopedic impairment that adversely affects the child's educational performance. The term includes impairments by congenital anomaly (e.g., club foot, absence of some member), impairments caused by some disease (e.g., poliomyelitis, bone tuberculosis), impairments from other causes (e.g., cerebral palsy, amputations), and fractures and burns that cause contractures.

VII. *Other health impaired* means limited strength, vitality, or alertness owing to chronic or acute health problems, such as a heart condition, tuberculosis, rheumatic fever, nephritis, asthma, sickle cell anemia, hemophilia, lead poisoning, leukemia, or diabetes, which adversely affect a child's educational performance.

VIII. *Seriously emotionally disturbed* is defined as follows:
   A. The term means a condition exhibiting one or more of the following characteristics over a long period of time which adversely affects educational performance:
      1. An inability to learn that cannot be explained by intellectual, sensory, or health factors
      2. An inability to build or maintain satisfactory interpersonal relationships with peers and teachers
      3. Inappropriate types of behavior or feelings under normal circumstances
      4. A general pervasive mood of unhappiness or depression
      5. A tendency to develop physical symptoms or fears associated with personal or school problems
IX. *Specific learning disability* means a disorder in one or more of the basic psychological processes involved in understanding or in using language, spoken or written, that may manifest itself in an imperfect ability to listen, think, speak, write, spell, or do mathematical calculations. The term includes children who have learning problems that are primarily the result of perceptual handicaps, brain injury, minimal brain dysfunction, dyslexia, and developmental aphasia. The term does not include children who have learning problems that are primarily the result of visual, hearing, or motor handicaps, or environmental, cultural, or economic disadvantages.
X. *Hearing impaired* means a communication disorder such as stuttering, impaired articulation, a language impairment, or a voice impairment that inhibits the child's educational performance.
XI. *Visually handicapped* means a visual impairment that, even with correction, adversely affects the child's educational performance. The term includes both partially seeing and blind children.

Not All Children with Disabilities Receive Special Education Services

Of special significance in meeting both letter and spirit of Public Law 101–476 is the Part (B) phrase "who, by reason thereof (i.e., of disability) need special education and related services." Part (B) ensures that special services, as determined by assessment, must be provided when necessary. However, it also ensures that the child cannot be subjected to a program that indiscriminately assigns her or him to that program simply because she or he has a disability (i.e., is mentally retarded, deaf, emotionally disturbed). Initially, assessment pursuant to Public Law 101–476 determines the type and extent of the individual's special needs, including needs in APE and TR. Subsequently, assessment determines to what extent special needs have yet to be met. Assessment further determines which educational environment(s) is best for each individual's special needs.

Pursuant to special education services called for in Part B above, Public Law 101–476 defines special education as follows:

> . . . specially designed instruction, at no cost to parents or guardians, to meet the unique needs of a child with a disability including:

(A) instruction conducted in the classroom, in the home, in hospitals and institutions, and in other settings; and

(B) instruction in physical education (PL 101–476, sec. 1401[a][16])

Related services are defined, in part, as follows:

. . . supportive services . . . including therapeutic recreation . . . as may be required to assist the child with disabilities to benefit from special education, and includes early identification and assessment of children with disabilities (PL 101–476, Sec. 602[a][17]).

Pursuant to the above excerpts from Public Law 101–476, services, including APE and TR, must be made available to eligible persons at no cost to parent or guardian. Further, these services must meet the individual's unique needs as identified through assessment, and must be provided in the least restrictive environment (LRE). *Least restrictive environment placement* is defined herein as placing the student with a disability at a point along a continuum of educational placement alternatives where all students, both with and without disabilities, coexist, interact, and learn to the fullest extent of each of their respective abilities. Proper placement (i.e., placement in the environment that is truly least restrictive for *all*) should not compromise the quality of learning for any student placed in that specific environment. The assessment process is perhaps the single most critical factor in determining whether educational placement is, truly, proper.

Who Determines Placement?

While Public Law 101–476 identifies and defines disabilities by name, it does not determine at the federal level which child with a defined disability actually receives special education services at the local level. This determination is left to the discretion of individual states and often to the individual school district. Definitions of disability as they appear in the *Federal Register* are open to rather wide interpretation. For example, the definition of mental retardation is couched in terms of "significantly subaverage intellectual functioning." The term deaf refers to any hearing impairment that "adversely affects educational performance." In each instance, and in similar instances in remaining categories, phrases such as "significantly subaverage" and "adversely affects" are open to interpretation. In some states, the state education agency leaves such interpretations to local discretion. APE and TR specialists must be thoroughly familiar with specific criteria to which their respective local and state education agencies adhere. Such criteria, regardless of where they originate, typically are referred to as program entry and exit criteria. These criteria provide the primary basis for determining at what educational levels the person is placed given the spectrum of placement alternatives. Knowledge of entry and exit criteria helps ensure that persons eligible for Public Law 101–476 services are assessed and, if found in need, receive appropriate, individualized APE or TR services.

Public Law 101–336 (Americans with Disabilities Act of 1990 [ADA])

Further assurance that persons with disabilities receive equitable service from *public* and *private* service providers comes from Public Law 101–336, the *Americans with*

Disabilities Act. This Act, passed in 1990, replaced and built upon its predecessor, Public Law 93–112, the *Rehabilitation Act of 1973* (Eichstaedt and Kalakian, 1993).

While Public Law 101–476 (IDEA) is a special education act, Public Law 101–336 (ADA) is a civil rights act. The latter mandates equal opportunity in facets of life including and beyond school.

Public Law 101–336 states, in part:

> . . . no qualified individual with a disability shall, solely by reason of such disability, be excluded from participation in or be denied the benefits of the services, programs, or activities of a public entity, or be subjected to discrimination by a public entity (Title II, Subtitle A, Sec. 202).

The law defines public entities as they have been traditionally defined, and further identifies the following private entities (among others) as public for purposes of the law:

> . . . a gymnasium, health spa, bowling alley, golf course, or other place of exercise or recreation (Title III, Sec. 301[7][A]).

In effect, the law provides that public and private institutions shall not discriminate against any person solely by reason of disability. Apropos to assessment and service provision in APE and TR, this law mandates that, in terms of receiving quality assessment-guided education in both public and private sectors, persons with disabilities must be given at least the same consideration afforded nondisabled peers.

Students Needing Adapted Physical Education or Therapeutic Recreation Services, but Who Are Not Eligible for Services Provided by Public Law 101–476 or Public Law 101–336

Aforementioned federal mandates are explicit in designating who is eligible to receive special services. These mandates, however, fall short of recognizing many persons who, though they do not meet various laws' definitions of disability, do have physical education and recreation needs that simply cannot be addressed meaningfully in the mainstream. For example, among such persons are those who, though not having disability by some legal definition, are obese or underdeveloped, have low fitness, are awkward or clumsy, or are temporarily (acutely) disabled. Such persons often are caught between individualized programs which they need but for which they do not qualify, and mainstream programs not capable of ensuring safe and successful participation. Since such persons are not eligible for services funded by special education, it is reasonable to assert that, in the interest of equal opportunity, such persons be meaningfully accommodated in regular, mainstream programs. Regular physical education and recreation specialists should be committed to identifying and meeting the needs of such persons.

The foregoing discussion of "Who are we assessing?" has described a wide range of characteristics of persons needing APE or TR services. APE and TR, as disciplines, are each unique in what they can do to enhance life quality among persons who have disabilities. These disciplines are also related in many ways. They are, indeed, allied services. There is great variance in types and degrees of disabilities and in ranges of physical, motor, social, and emotional needs among persons to be served. Tremendous differences among persons who could benefit from APE and TR services demand that well-trained professionals in APE and TR cooperate, network, and share expertise. A true team cooperation spirit among allied professionals will help ensure (1) thorough assessment, (2) comprehensive interpretation of assessment data, and (3) provision of individualized service drawn from the full spectrum of available service options.

Any final analysis of who we *must* assess comes down to who the mandates require that we assess. However, concern only with who, by mandate, must be assessed leaves these writers with feelings best characterized as cold and impersonal. True concern, in the committed, professional sense, should be for who *should* we assess. While the "pat" answer might be everyone, a more realistic and practical answer is anyone who might reasonably be expected to benefit from a suitably modified APE or TR experience.

Zero Reject and Zero Fail

Answering the question "Who ought to be assessed?" can be best facilitated when we address the concepts of zero reject and zero fail (Eichstaedt, 1991). First, virtually every student well enough to receive a formal education must be considered entitled to some form of physical education or recreation, however modified. Physical educators and recreators, especially APE and TR specialists, must strive to meet needs of every person for whom their school or agency is responsible. This is *zero reject*. Second, students/clients should not and need not fail in physical education and recreation programs when providers address each person's unique needs and capabilities. In this context, physical education and recreation can facilitate the goal of *zero fail* by building in success.

We must be committed to identifying students/clients who, for whatever reason and at any given time, are not capable of safely and successfully participating in mainstream programs. Our challenge is to advocate for *all* persons that they might enjoy enhanced life quality through physical education and recreation. Our responsibility in our respective (APE and TR) disciplines is to identify the unique strengths and needs of each individual and develop strategies that enable her or him to achieve life quality according to potential. We should strive to accentuate the positive, focus on ability rather than disability, and select strategies that minimize whatever limitations the disability might be placing on individual achievement.

References

Eichstaedt, C. B. "Adapted Physical Education: A State of the Art." Paper presented at the annual meeting of the Illinois Association for Health, Physical Education, Recreation, and Dance, November 1991.

Eichstaedt, C. B., and L. H. Kalakian. *Developmental/Adapted Physical Education: Making Ability Count,* 3rd ed. New York: Macmillan, 1993.

Federal Register. "Final Regulations of the Education for All Handicapped Children Act, Implementation of Part B of the Education of the Handicapped Act." Department of Health, Education, and Welfare, Office of Education, vol. 42(163), Part II, August 23, 1977, Section 121a5, Special Education, 42478.

Public Law 93–112. (1973). *Rehabilitation Act of 1973.* Section 504, Title V, 23.

Public Law 99–457. (1986, October 8). *Education of the Handicapped Act Amendments of 1986.* (99th Congress, 2nd session, House of Representatives, Report 99–995).

Public Law 101–336. (1990, July 26). *Americans with Disabilities Act of 1990.* Title II, Subtitle A, Section 202.

IBID. Title III, Section 301(7)(A).

Public Law 101–476. (1990, October 30). *Individuals with Disabilities Education Act.* Section 1401(a)(1).

IBID. Section 1401(a)(16).

IBID. Section 602(a)(17).

Stein, J. U. "The Mission and the Mandate: Physical Education, the Not So Sleeping Giant." *Education Unlimited,* 6, June 1979.

CHAPTER 2

Why Are We Assessing?

When an APE or TR specialist scrutinizes information derived from testing and measuring student/client ability, he or she is engaging in assessment. Technically, a test is nothing more than a method for gathering information. Measurements are the data one derives from administering tests. Assessment refers specifically to the specialist's *interpretation* of measures obtained through testing. Seaman and DePauw (1989, p. 131) define assessment as "interpreting the measurements for the purpose of making decisions about placement, program planning, and performance objectives." Assessment is the critical link in the testing process that renders worthwhile the time spent gathering data. Assessment also provides the basis for what instruction should follow.

Test results, by themselves, do not translate into programs for students/clients. Test results are data; nothing more, nothing less. The real value of data is determined solely by the specialist's ability to interpret data. From these interpretations (i.e., assessments), an individual's needs can be identified, and the APE or TR specialist can begin to fashion programs and experiences designed to meet individual needs.

Assessment: The Legal Obligation

Assessment lies at the very heart of individualizing APE and TR experiences for persons who have disabilities. In many instances, assessment is required by law. While state laws regarding assessment vary, certain federal mandates are universally applicable.

As mentioned in Chapter One, development of individualized learning experiences in the least restrictive environment is the cornerstone of Public Law 101–476 (*Individuals with Disabilities Education Act of 1990* [IDEA]). Services mandated by IDEA, including comprehensive assessment, cover all persons with disabilities ages 3–21. IDEA, though it does not require special services for infants and toddlers ages 0–2, strongly recommends that such services be provided. Rationale behind the assessment sections of the mandate is founded in logic that individualized instruction is possible only when one knows the individual, and one cannot know the individual without assessment.

Need for assessment also is implied in Public Law 101–336 (*Americans with Disabilities Act of 1990*) to the extent that any agency receiving federal funds must not discriminate against any person solely by virtue of disability. Pursuant to this mandate, persons with disabilities must be afforded programs of at least the same quality as are those provided for persons without disabilities. Here, assessment becomes a key component in fulfilling both letter and spirit of this mandate.

Assessment: The Moral Obligation

Among the principles for which any great society stands is equal opportunity for all members. Equal opportunity becomes each member's inalienable right.

This premise is not always practiced. Persons with disabilities, particularly those with special needs, have often borne much of the brunt of educational and social inequity. Historically, persons with disabilities have been the last to receive services when times become good and first to lose services when times become bad. Reasons for inequities have ranged from intentional inaction to benign neglect. Advocates of full enfranchisement for persons with disabilities have had to lobby intensely for special legislation, and have looked to the courts for assurance that such legislation, once passed, is heeded.

Assessment for Screening Purposes

Screening is a process by which persons potentially in need of special services are initially identified. Screening must be considered an integral component of any comprehensive assessment program. Screening measures usually are rather cursory in nature and relatively easy to administer. Typically, time devoted to screening per participant is not protracted.

Screening is part of a first line of defense that helps determine whether further, in-depth diagnostic procedures need to be ordered. Screening is proactive, because its goal is early identification of persons with special needs who might benefit from special services.

Screening tests, unlike more thorough diagnostic tests, generally require no special permission from parents or guardians to be administered. Only when specific persons are singled out for special testing is it necessary to secure permission to test. Instruments termed screening devices generally are routinely administered to all members of a group. Whenever a test is routine and administered universally, no special permission to test a given person is required.

Screening serves at least two important purposes: (1) it can help confirm or allay concerns regarding a student's/client's developmental status, and (2) it can aid in identification of those whose special needs have, heretofore, gone unnoticed.

Typically the most effective (including cost effective) intervention is early intervention. Screening's primary goal should be early identification of special needs to facilitate appropriate interventions as soon as possible.

Assessment for Diagnostic Purposes

Screening is only the beginning of an assessment process that determines what APE or TR needs might exist. Persons who meet screening criteria should be referred for further, in-depth diagnostic assessment. Here, permission must be sought from the parent or guardian prior to initiating further, new diagnostic, testing. Assessment at this level helps determine precisely what special needs exist and how those needs might most effectively be met. Thorough diagnostic assessment provides a basis for in-depth determination of the individual's unique needs and for fashioning programs designed specifically to meet those needs.

In educational settings, responsibility for diagnostic assessment typically rests with a team of persons that includes the following:

1. The child's current classroom teacher
2. The child's special education teacher
3. A representative of the school administration
4. The child's parent or guardian
5. The child (when appropriate)
6. Other persons mutually agreed upon by the above (e.g., physical therapist, occupational therapist, neurologist, orthopedist, recreational therapist, adapted physical education specialist)

Assessment to Secure Program Funding

Funding to provide special services to persons who have disabilities must be justified. Such economic reality faces virtually all program and service providers, and assessment is central to any funding justification process. Assessment must determine not only numbers of persons needing service, but types of services needed. This is particularly true among public agencies where formulae subsequently are applied to numbers; and funding, to the extent available, follows. For example, funding for Public Law 101–476-related APE and TR services comes, in part, from federal tax dollars. These dollars are designated as *pass through* dollars. Pass through is the procedure by which federal dollars for special services pass *from* the federal government, *through* state government, *to* local government. In each instance, dollar flow is based on demonstrated (i.e., assessment determined) need.

Assessment to Determine Curriculum/Program Effectiveness

Anyone who provides services to people, be they students, clients, participants, or customers, must have some basis for determining if a program in question is, indeed, functioning effectively. Program evaluation is an essential ingredient in any service provision model because it asks the essential question, "Is the program fulfilling its purpose?" Seaman and DePauw (1989) cite three essential assessment considerations in program evaluation: (1) the learning environment, (2) the learners, and (3) learning.

Assessing the Learning Environment

Given the scope of this text, learning environment assessment is not the major emphasis. Rather, focus will be on the learner and the learning that takes place. Assessment of the learning environment is, nonetheless, important. It addresses considerations such as facilities, quantity and quality of equipment and supplies, staff competence, and support for the program. For example, is a therapy pool available? Does everyone needing a specific equipment item have that item at his or her disposal when necessary? Is equipment in a good state of repair? Do staff members hold recognized licenses or certifications? What is the student-to-teacher ratio? Answers to these questions clearly impact program quality.

Assessing the Learners

Aforementioned mandates and professional obligation require that the assessment of learners be central to any process that individualizes instruction. One must first know the learner before one can meaningfully determine what learning should take place. However, coming to know the learner as a unique individual can be a process replete with pitfalls.

Knowledge of a learner's disability alone (e.g., spina bifida, cerebral palsy) does virtually nothing to facilitate the APE or TR specialist's understanding of that learner's unique APE or TR needs. APE and TR specialists must clearly understand that a learner's disability is but one part (often not the most critical part) of a whole person, and that sometimes there is a tendency, even among some professionals, to focus unduly on the disability.

Provision of service founded in emphasis on learner disability disserves both the learner and the profession. First, the approach is negative, tending to focus on what the learner cannot do rather than can do. The net result typically is programming characterized by lowered expectations for persons being served. Unfortunately, lowered expectations typically become self-fulfilling prophecies. Second, this approach promotes the critically misleading notion that all persons with the same disability (i.e., label; for example, mental disability) have the same needs. Assessment helps avoid this pitfall, because it enables seeing the learner as a unique individual, as well as enabling determination of the learner's true needs irrespective of label. For example, if two people with cerebral palsy participate in the same program, it must be because their respective needs and interests are similar, not because their labels are the same. Respect for the learner's uniqueness must remain paramount, and assessment to reveal that uniqueness is critical to learner-centered (rather than label-centered) program development.

Assessing Learning

Once the learner's unique needs have been identified, a program can be tailored to meet those needs. Obviously, any program designed to meet needs is not complete unless procedures are in place to determine whether needs identified have been met. At this juncture, assessment becomes the process that determines the degree to which the learner has, in fact, learned.

Recognizing that learning has occurred is as important for the learner and parent as it is for the APE or TR specialist. Awareness of entry level status followed by knowledge of improvement is motivating to any person able to conceptualize the significance of improvement. When realistic goals are set and assessment provides evidence of progress, achievement from the learner's vantage point becomes concrete. Concomitant outcomes of the learner's knowledge of achievement often include improved self-esteem and heightened motivation.

Progress assessments are essential for parents/guardians so they can know the extent of their child's achievements. Concerned parents/guardians desire the best learning opportunities for their children, and assessments of learning help parents judge improvement.

Among parents of children with disabilities, two progress-related assessment inquiries usually emerge. On one hand, parents want to know the extent of achievement according to the child's potential. On the other hand, they desire to know their child's educational status and progress relative to peers without disabilities. Finally, if parents are to assume a meaningful role as partners in facilitating their child's development, they must have a basis (i.e., assessment results) for determining effectiveness of present interventions.

Assessment to Determine How the Person with Disability's Performance Compares with Other Persons Having a Similar Disability (Norm-Referenced Tests)

One dictum in norm-referenced assessment is that norms, with few exceptions, should be applied to a student/client only if persons similar to that student/client were represented in the group from which the norms were developed. In other words, if a person has a mental disability, norms to which that person is compared should have been derived from performance scores of other persons with similar mental disabilities. A limited number of norm-referenced tests for persons who have disabilities are available. Examples include: Physical Fitness and Motor Skill Levels of Individuals with Mental Retardation: Mild, Moderate, and Down Syndrome, Ages 6–21 (Eichstaedt et al., 1991); Physical Fitness Testing of the Disabled [norms for persons who have visual impairments, auditory impairments, cerebral palsy, spinal neuromuscular conditions, congenital anomalies, and acquired amputations] (Winnick and Short, 1985); Motor Fitness Testing Manual for the Mildly Mentally Retarded (AAHPERD, 1976a); and Motor Fitness Testing Manual for the

Moderately Mentally Retarded (AAHPERD, 1976b). The latter two instruments are offered for informational purposes only. Norms are no longer current, and technical adequacy might be questionable.

Assessment to Determine Departure from Typical Development (Norm-Referenced Tests)

At times, it is legitimate, even essential, to compare a person whose development is known or believed to be delayed to that of persons whose development is known to be typical. The purpose of such assessment is to determine if the development of the person with the disability departs sufficiently from the norm to warrant provision of special services. Typically, opportunity to participate in special programs is contingent upon the person's meeting *entry criteria* for participation in the given program. For example, an entry criterion might be a score falling two standard deviations below the mean on a standardized, norm-referenced test. A person scoring below two standard deviations below the mean would, by that criterion at least, qualify for special services.

Because norm-referenced tests compare the individual's performance to an established standard (i.e., the norm), such tests can be particularly helpful in determining (1) if a person with a disability qualifies for special service, and (2) if so, at what level. The following norm-referenced tests, while normed on typically developing populations, are examples of tests often used in making placement decisions for persons with disabilities: Bruininks-Oseretsky Test of Motor Proficiency (Bruininks, 1978) and Battelle Developmental Inventory (Newborg, Stock, and Wnek, 1984). These tests are cited as examples only, but are cited particularly because their authors considered needs and attributes of persons with disabilities in their respective test development processes.

One caveat when using norm-referenced tests to assess persons with disabilities is that a norm-referenced test designed for use with typically developing populations might unfairly discriminate against the person with the disability. For example, a shuttle run designed to measure agility in mainstream students may, instead, measure intelligence in mentally retarded students. It is important to note that entry criteria, in addition to standardized (norm-referenced) test scores, likely will be in place for diagnostic assessment purposes, and that the person being assessed likely will be required also to meet other entry criteria for special program placement.

Assessment to Determine Development According to Some Set Criterion (Criterion-Referenced Tests)

Often there is a need to determine a person's individual status with respect to some specific skill or behavior. Here, the person is compared to predesignated performance or behavior criteria. This is termed *criterion-referenced assessment*. With criterion-referenced assessment, the person is not being compared to others. For example, the teacher/leader might identify four developmentally sequenced stages through which a person progresses in achieving a mature overhand throw. Each stage may be identified, and a criterion statement for each can be written in objectively measurable (behavioral) terms. The teacher/leader then observes the person executing the overhand throw, and determines which performance criteria, if any, the person already has achieved. Performance criteria yet to be achieved, once identified, can provide direction for future instructional strategies.

Criterion-referenced assessments can be particularly helpful when determining what to do once the student/client has been placed in a special program. Once the decision has been made that a specific skill ought to be the focus of a student's/client's program, criterion-referenced assessment becomes helpful in two very important ways. First, it determines the student's/client's stage of development with respect to the skill in question. Second, it reveals the subsequent stage of development for that skill, which then becomes the focus of instruction.

Assessment to Determine Appropriate Placement

Delivery of APE or TR services should occur along a continuum of placement alternatives. Successful placement at any point along the continuum has been achieved when *all* learners/participants in that particular setting have meaningful opportunity to achieve their respective potentials. Services should be provided in a setting that is as normalizing and near the mainstream as possible. Depending on the individual and the activity in question, a participant's placement along this continuum may vary. In some instances, the individual may safely and successfully participate in or near the mainstream. In others, the individual might best be served in a setting apart from the mainstream. At minimum, two criteria need be invoked to determine if participant placement at any level along the continuum is appropriate. First, placement of an individual with a disability in any given setting should not compromise the quality of that individual's experience in that setting. Second, that individual's placement in any given setting must not compromise the experience of other persons with or without disabilities who are also in that setting.

Possible placement alternatives ranging from least to most restrictive environment in school settings are as follows:

LEVEL 1. Full-time placement in the regular setting

LEVEL 2. Full-time integrated placement in the regular program, but with consultation, as needed, between regular teacher/leader and APE or TR specialist (may include peer tutors, cross-age tutors, and reverse mainstreaming)

LEVEL 3. Part-time placement in the regular setting; part time placement in a modified setting apart from the mainstream

LEVEL 4. Full-time placement in a modified setting apart from the mainstream (regular school)

LEVEL 5. Full-time placement in a modified setting apart from the mainstream (nonresidential, special school)

LEVEL 6. Full-time placement in a modified setting apart from the mainstream (residential, special school)

Placement alternatives for persons participating in physical education or recreation activities outside of school settings will depend primarily upon the breadth of options available at a given time and in a given place. In both school and nonschool settings, a program's success should be assessed, at least in part, by numbers of participants with disabilities effectively screened into, rather than out of, mainstream programs. The goal should be to place the person as close to the school mainstream and typical community setting as is effectively possible. Often, norm-referenced tests will be relied upon significantly in determining which placement alternative will best suit the individual.

References

American Alliance for Health, Physical Education, Recreation, and Dance. *Motor Fitness Testing Manual for the Mildly Mentally Retarded.* Washington, D.C.: The Alliance, 1976a.

American Alliance for Health, Physical Education, Recreation, and Dance. *Motor Fitness Testing Manual for the Moderately Mentally Retarded.* Washington, D.C.: The Alliance, 1976b.

Bruininks, R. *Bruininks-Oseretsky Test of Motor Proficiency.* Circle Pines, MN: American Guidance Service, 1978.

Eichstaedt, C. B., P. Y. Wang, J. J. Polacek, and P. F. Dohrmann. *Physical Fitness and Motor Skill Levels of Individuals with Mental Retardation: Mild, Moderate, and Down Syndrome, Ages 6–21.* Normal, IL: Illinois State University Printing Services, 1991.

Newborg, J., J. R. Stock, and L. Wnek. *Battelle Developmental Inventory.* Allen, TX: Developmental Learning Resources, 1984.

Public Law 101–336. (1990, July 26). *Americans with Disabilities Act.* 101st Congress.

Public Law 101–476. (1990, October 30). *Individuals with Disabilities Education Act.* 101st Congress.

Seaman, J. A., and K. P. DePauw. *The New Adapted Physical Education: A Developmental Approach,* 2nd ed. Mountain View, CA: Mayfield, 1989.

Winnick, J. P., and F. X. Short. *Physical Fitness Testing of the Disabled: Project UNIQUE.* Champaign, IL: Human Kinetics, 1985.

CHAPTER 3

Getting to Know the Student/Client

Any proficiency demonstrated by the student/client today is one that has been shaped by events that make up his or her growth and development history. When assessing performance in any domain, determining performance levels within that domain marks but one phase of the assessment process. The APE and TR specialist conducting any comprehensive assessment must also understand factors that have helped shape the current performance. Environmental enrichment or deprivation, deleterious or traumatic events, and physical and sensory impairments are but a few historical factors that may have affected the student's/client's present level of function. Once a student/client has been referred for APE or TR assessment, the tester must become a "detective" who gathers relevant historical as well as current information. Armed with both current and historical information, the APE or TR specialist will invariably be better positioned to understand and plan for the person's adapted physical education or recreation future. Knowing where the student/client has come from (i.e., her or his life experience) virtually always facilitates insights into how the student/client has arrived at the present. These insights, in turn, help lay the foundation for selecting strategies most likely to facilitate the student's/client's achieving her or his potential.

Getting to know the student/client is a process that begins not with selecting and administering tests, but with the assessor's going back to the student's/client's beginnings. Such beginnings, to the extent records are available, are found in health and medical records, psychological work-ups, school files, case studies, and anecdotal reports.

Health-Related Records

To plan an appropriate adapted physical education or therapeutic recreation program, the teacher/leader must scrutinize available health and medical records for relevant information. At the outset of this discussion, it is essential for APE or TR specialists to understand clearly that such records are confidential and must always be treated as such. In both school and agency settings, the nurse or other health personnel can assist in reviewing available records for a particular student/client. Health and medical files should be examined for essential information including, though not necessarily limited to, the following:

1. Chronic or acute illnesses (e.g., diabetes, chronic heart condition, chronic asthma)
2. Sensory impairments (e.g., vision or hearing loss, speech or language difficulties)
3. Physical impairments (cerebral palsy, muscular dystrophy, amputation)
4. Record of mild illnesses (e.g., frequency of colds, headaches, stomachaches) and records of absenteeism due to illness
5. Names of physicians and therapists
6. Written permission from parent/guardian to contact medical personnel in case of emergency
7. Phone numbers of parents/guardians in case of emergency
8. Medications and their purposes

A quick perusal of a student's health file can be valuable because it often reveals vital historical information about the person's health history. This preliminary assessment may pinpoint areas in need of further assessment. For example, a health file may indicate that Amy receives physical therapy once per week. It is crucial that the APE or TR specialist determine reasons for and the nature of the therapy. Such information enables the teacher or therapist to provide Amy with experiences that help facilitate her physical therapy goals. This situation, likewise, should work equally in reverse. For example, appropriate physical therapy may be prescribed to facilitate Amy's achieving her recreation and physical education potential.

Before obtaining information from a therapist, physician, or other allied health professional, it is essential to follow due process procedures and secure parent/guardian permission for the student's/client's records to be released. Following release of the student's/client's records and the APE or TR specialist's perusal of such, the APE or TR specialist will come to better know the student/client. At this juncture, it may be appropriate for the specialist to contact the parent/guardian, physician, school or agency nurse, and other therapists and allied health personnel whose names appear in the file. With the file providing an important information base, the APE or TR specialist can engage the aforementioned allied professionals in dialog that more fully reveals the student's/client's history, current status, and future needs. It is equally important that the APE or TR specialist relate (as well as receive) information about the student/client to the aforementioned specialists. Information from the APE or TR specialist will be beneficial to others in the health care network to the extent that they will come to see the student/client from the APE or TR specialist's unique perspective.

The APE or TR specialist, along with allied professionals, the parent/guardian, and the student/client (when appropriate), must work cooperatively to plan an appropriate program based on assessment information from many sources. It is important that each of the above be involved in assessing and planning, because each sees the student/client from his or her unique perspective. Sometimes there is the tendency for one specialist, if acting in relative isolation from allied specialists, to see the student/client only through the eyes of his or her specialty. Generally, the more perspectives available, the greater the likelihood the student/client will be perceived and subsequently served as a whole person. This "whole person" approach helps reveal a wide spectrum of abilities; abilities often interrelated and interdependent. Finally, the more comprehensively individual needs are identified, the greater the likelihood that individual needs can be met and program objectives achieved. Table 3.1 presents a sample form that can be used to gather activity-related information about a student/client. This specific form solicits information from the student's/client's physician.

When seeking historical information about the student/client, particular attention should be paid to the following:

1. Medical diagnosis
2. Condition's severity
3. Prognosis
4. Psychological evaluations
5. Symptoms or characteristics relative to their potential for impact in adapted physical education and therapeutic recreation settings
6. Past and current courses of treatment
7. Recommended activities (source, rationale)
8. Restricted activities (source, rationale)
9. Telephone numbers of parents/guardians
10. Telephone numbers of previously or currently attending physicians and other allied professionals

APE and TR specialists who attempt to secure information from physicians about their students/clients need to be aware that, for a variety of reasons, such information may not always be immediately forthcoming. Difficulty (sometimes frustrations) encountered in communicating with physicians, however, in no way absolves APE or TR specialists from responsibility to secure essential information as needed.

The physician may respond slowly and often cautiously for a variety of reasons. How soon or thoroughly a physician responds may depend, in part, on how highly the physician prioritizes the APE or TR specialist's need for information. Some physicians, concerned about medical malpractice in a society that has become overly litigious, are hesitant to provide information that could become the basis for future litigation. At this point it is fair to emphasize that for the same reason a physician may be hesitant to provide information, it may be equally important for the APE or TR specialist to have information. Finally, physicians are bound by confidentiality, and the physician's willingness to respond will be better ensured when he or she has written permission from a parent/guardian to share patient history with the APE or TR specialist.

TABLE 3.1 Sample Medical Information Form (Minnesota Developmental/
Adapted Physical Education, Region 11E, 1981)

MEDICAL AUTHORIZATION FORM
LONG-TERM DISABILITY

REGION 11E

DATE SENT: _____ Minnesota Developmental/Adapted Physical Education

Minnesota State Law requires that all students participate in physical education on a regular basis. If a permanent or long-term disability interferes with participation in the regular physical education program, an individualized physical education curriculum will be planned around the student's motor strengths and abilities. The student shall be enrolled in the *adapted program* based on completion of this form.

Student's Name _____ D.O.B. _____ School _____ Grade _____

Parent/Guardian _____ Phone _____

Disability _____

_____

Expected Duration of Disability _____

Medication (implication for physical activity) _____

_____

The following activities will be adapted to the student's individual capabilities. Please check any activity you would **NOT** recommend for the above student.

I. Physical Fitness Activities
_____ arm-shoulder strength
_____ abdominal strength
_____ flexibility (range of motion)
_____ cardio-respiratory endurance
_____ leg strength

II. Locomotor Activities
_____ creeping
_____ crawling
_____ walking
_____ running
_____ sliding
_____ hopping
_____ jumping
_____ skipping
_____ galloping

III. Non-Locomotor Activities
_____ bending   _____ hanging
_____ twisting   _____ balancing
_____ pushing   _____ swinging
_____ pulling
_____ lifting

IV. Aquatics
_____ swimming skills
_____ water play
_____ diving

V. Object Control Skills
_____ catching
_____ kicking
_____ striking
_____ overhand throwing
_____ underhand throwing
_____ ball bouncing

VI. Other Activities Not Recommended:
_____
_____
_____
_____
_____
_____
_____
_____
_____
_____
_____

COMMENTS: _____

_____

_____

Your input will assist us in determining an appropriate instructional program.

Date: _____   Signed: _____ , M.D.

Phone Number: _____

Psychological Work-Ups

If the person about to be tested is in a school or agency setting, there is a likelihood that the person may have been referred previously for assessment to a school or agency psychologist. Such assessments, both formal and informal, can provide insights that help the current tester understand how the student's/client's psychological characteristics might have been, in part, responsible for his or her current performance status. These considerations might also facilitate decisions regarding types of tests that need to be administered and, respecting test standardization procedures, under what environmental conditions said tests most likely would yield reliable and valid information. Finally, understanding the student's/client's psychological frame of reference can facilitate selection of interventions with greatest potential to ensure future success in any program.

School Files

Another valuable information source for facilitating comprehensive adapted physical education and therapeutic recreation assessment and program development is the student's cumulative school file. These files are established for each student when she or he first enters school, and "follow" the student through school until graduation. While precise content of cumulative records varies among school districts, there has been a trend recently to remove subjective reports and include only objective information. Once the student/client has been referred for assessment, the tester should examine the student's/client's cumulative file. Generally, homeroom teachers and school guidance counselors will have access to the cumulative file for each student to whom they are assigned. Cumulative files typically include the following:

1. Student's name and address
2. Name and address of parent/guardian
3. Family status (siblings and ages)
4. Emergency contact person
5. Standardized achievement test scores
6. General school progress reports
7. Schoolwork samples (sometimes)
8. Photograph of student

Another source of historical information available from the school setting is the student's special education file. For every student identified as having a disability, there should be a special education record on file. Special education files can provide a wealth of critical information including the following:

1. Primary disability and when diagnosed
2. Severity of disability (level of special education services provided in the past)
3. Family status (siblings and ages)

4. All special education services provided currently and in the past, including names of service providers
5. Previous individualized education programs (IEPs)
6. Records of progress toward IEP short-term objectives and long-term goals
7. All due process and permission forms

Special education files can be extremely valuable in planning an adapted physical education or therapeutic recreation plan of action. Say, for example, the student's special education file reveals a history of distractability and severe learning disability. Such information can most certainly help guide the tester in deciding what types of tests to administer and under what conditions (respecting standardization procedures, of course) such tests should be administered. Yet another source of valuable first-hand information is the student's special education teacher who can reveal insights often not quantifiable or objectively measurable.

The Client's Agency File

Whenever a client has historically been served by a particular agency, that agency typically will maintain records of that client's participation. Often, the kinds of information found in health-related records and school and special education files will be reflected in agency files. Depending upon the nature of the service provided by the particular agency, information specific to that agency's program emphasis will appear in the file. If the client has completed participation in a given agency's program, the tester presently can review pretest results, progress reports, and posttest results recorded during the client's participation in that agency's program. Of particular value will be insights from summary reports and anecdotal reporting. Such reporting often affords information not revealable when reviewing numbers alone. One caveat, however, in reviewing any subjective information is that such information might be colored by personal biases and/or professional competence of the previous reporter. This caveat is particularly germane when the current tester, reading subjective information from a client's previous agency file, has little or no knowledge of the person(s) who have entered subjective information into that file.

Insights from Parents/Guardians

Parents/guardians have the right to be involved in their child's assessment, and should be involved in various ways besides those required by legal mandates. Parents/guardians can play an essential assessment role by reporting information, typically from a naturalistic setting, about their child's history. Once a child has been referred for APE or TR assessment, parents/guardians should be contacted for information about the child's developmental history, including interviews and/or complete case histories. Often, the kind of information revealed by parents/guardians is known only by parents, since school or agency personnel may have little or no knowledge of the student's past, and typically observe behavior only within the context of the program in which the student/client is enrolled.

Seaman and DePauw (1989) offer a format for facilitating case studies resulting from dialog with parents/guardians. Selections from this format may serve as a guide for professionals interviewing parents/guardians. The format, with some modification, is as follows:

Background information—child's/student's/client's name and birth date, parent's/guardian's names, siblings (including age and gender)

Prenatal and natal history—length of pregnancy, pregnancy history, birth weight, notable conditions occurring during and immediately following birth

Physical and developmental history—health history, present health status, history of developmental milestones' appearances (e.g., sitting, walking, toileting, talking)

Social and personal development—friend relationships, sibling relationships, hobby and recreational interests (including what the person might be interested in if given opportunity), attitudes towards parents/ guardians, home, school, agency

School/agency participation history—summary of school and agency experiences, current performance levels, history of progress towards current performance levels, test scores and dates (including interpretations of tests), teachers'/therapists'/allied professionals' reports, current program content (including IEP, if available)

Interviews, in particular, must be conducted with sensitivity. The interviewer must encourage the parent/guardian to talk freely, while minimizing, to the extent feasible, his or her own participation. The interview's purpose should be made clear to the parent/guardian. This will facilitate the parent's/guardian's ability to reveal essential, focused insights. Interview questions should reflect the interview's focus and be objective, for example, "At what age did Andy walk?" One example of an inappropriately (subjectively) phrased question would be "Andy did walk by age 1, didn't he?" Questions couched in subjectivity can sometimes lead to respondent defensiveness, and this, in turn, compromises the likelihood of conducting a productive interview. Table 3.2 suggests a useful format for interviewing parent's/ guardian's about their child's/ward's motor development history.

Insights from Other School/Agency Personnel

Further valuable information sources in getting to know a student/client are teachers other than those previously cited. These sources are particularly valuable if the student/client, previously in a regular (i.e., unmodified) program, has only recently been referred for APE or TR assessment. These coworkers will be able to offer insights that shed light on how the current referral for assessment came to be deemed necessary. Mainstream classroom teachers, speech clinicians, and physical educators may be able to share observations about a student's motor development, fitness, and general behavioral and play behavior history. Such historical information can be most helpful if it has been systematically recorded cumulatively and in

TABLE 3.2 Suggested Format for Interviewing Parents or Guardians about the Child's Motor Development History

---

Parent Interview
Adapted Physical Education
Gross Motor Development

Interview

Student _____ ➤ _____ Date _____

Date of Birth _____ Grade/Teacher _____

Interviewer _____

Name of Parent/Guardian _____

Address _____ Phone _____

_____

	YES	NO	UNSURE
_____ (Child's Name)			
A. Motor Development			
1. First walked without crawling beforehand (creeping on hands and knees)			
2. First walked before 12 months			
3. First walked between 12–18 months			
4. First walked between 18–24 months			
5. First walked after 24 months			
6. Seemed to sit, stand, and walk late			
7. Walks on toes			
8. Walks flat-footed			
B. Coordination			
9. Falls frequently			
10. Bumps into things, people frequently			
11. Loses balance easily			
12. Seems to show shaky, jerky movements			
C. Body Awareness			
13. Feels uncomfortable about his or her body			
14. Confused easily about directions (e.g., right, left, forward, sideways)			
15. Understands basic body parts and their relationships (e.g., front, back, arm, foot)			
D. Physical Fitness			
16. Tires easily			
17. Overweight			
18. Seems to lack strength			
19. Lacks vitality (energy, enthusiasm)			
E. Social and Emotional Development			
20. Enjoys balls, bats, and other movement toys (jump ropes, rebounder)			
21. Plays outdoors often			
22. Plays vigorously with other children			
23. Enjoys gym class			
24. Participates in extracurricular physical activities			
25. Enjoys playing physical games and sports			

chronological order. When such information has been recorded, patterns of behavior, growth, and development become more apparent. Historical information from school/agency personnel may be gathered through interviews or by use of other informal measures including rating scales or checklists.

Other school personnel who may provide valuable preassessment information to the APE or TR specialist include nurses, administrators, teacher aides, and occupational therapists. The school nurse, in particular, might share information not always found in a student's school file. Often, the school nurse will have had meetings or conversations with the student's parents, physician, or other therapists. Although essential information usually is documented in the health file, insights, opinions, and judgments of aforementioned personnel should not be ignored. Indeed, they should be weighed along with other informal assessment information.

Nonschool personnel from whom valuable information may be gathered include agency activity leaders, nurses, social workers, and administrators. In addition, if the person lives in a group home, the group home supervisor may shed light on the individual's needs. Finally, if the person to be assessed currently is or has been employed, her or his employment supervisor or the personnel director may provide important insights from the workplace perspective.

Insights from the Student/Client

Too often, the student/client is overlooked or under-utilized as a valuable source of information. The student/client able to comprehend questions regarding his or her interests, needs, and developmental history might well be the single most valuable source of information. Sometimes, however, because of handicapism (as with other "isms") the person with a disability is not perceived by persons without disabilities as being particularly capable of determining and articulating her or his own unique interests and needs. APE and TR specialists need to recognize this "ism," and, when appropriate, go directly to the student/client for information typically solicited from others. Any question asked of someone else about the student/client is a question that, when appropriate, should be addressed directly to the student/client.

When meeting a student/client initially for the purpose of getting to know him or her, effort to establish rapport at the meeting's outset is essential. Rapport helps alleviate anxiety on the student's/client's part that might otherwise restrict the flow of important information. During the process of establishing rapport, it is important that the student/client know the purpose of the meeting. For example, the interviewer might say, "I've asked you to meet with me this morning to share with you what our program has to offer. Just as important, our staff is genuinely interested in what you would like to learn and do as you participate in our program." When interviewing children or persons whose social and/or mental ages do not roughly equate with chronological ages, communications should be geared to the individual's developmental status.

Who Assesses What?

Interpretation of test data provides a major means of getting to know the student/client. Yet, historically, there has not always been clear determination or agreement among allied professionals regarding who assesses what. Physical education and leisure assessments of persons with disabilities historically have been undertaken by persons other than APE and TR personnel. It is not particularly uncommon for persons with disabilities to have been assessed for physical education and leisure purposes by regular physical education and recreation personnel, occupational therapists, physical therapists, corrective therapists, mainstream classroom teachers, special education teachers, and sometimes psychologists. Suffice it to say that *anyone* who conducts physical education and leisure assessments among persons with disabilities *must* be thoroughly familiar with the test, test content, and test administration procedures. Standard operating procedure for any given school or agency should mandate that persons conducting adapted physical education and/or therapeutic recreation assessments be firmly grounded in these respective discipline specialties.

At times, there will be *honest* differences of opinion among allied professionals regarding who assesses what. For example, flexibility is one component of physical fitness, and, as such, is typically addressed in a physical education curriculum. Flexibility, likewise, is addressed in physical therapy. The occupational therapist may assess throwing, because throwing is perceived by the therapist to be a manipulative skill. Yet, the same skill might be assessed by an adapted physical education or therapeutic recreation specialist, because each respectively sees throwing skill development as being within the purview of her or his own profession.

Often, there are not clear cut boundaries for determining if a given activity belongs to a specific profession. This perhaps is as it should be, since professionals who worry more about territorial imperatives than students/clients may be putting their professions ahead of the very persons whom the professions are trying to serve. Allied professionals who serve the same student/client must strive to create a working environment characterized by two-way communication, mutual respect, and, foremost, mutual concern for best interests of the person being served.

Assessment by the Physical Educator

Physical education teachers are involved in assessment at a variety of levels. The elementary physical educator may be responsible for conducting initial *screening* at preschool or kindergarten age levels. Screening is a type of general assessment administered to all students in a class. At early age levels, motor screening becomes part of a larger, more comprehensive screening of general cognitive, affective, psychological, and social development. Children diagnosed as having disabilities at early age levels are usually referred for more in-depth diagnostic assessment.

The physical educator may also conduct screening tests at primary and upper elementary grade levels. General fitness tests, like the AAHPERD Youth Fitness Test (AAHPERD, 1976), AAHPERD Health Related Fitness Test

(AAHPERD, 1980), historically have been administered at elementary through secondary levels. According to AAHPERD today, Physical Best now replaces all previously endorsed AAHPERD tests (AAHPERD, 1988). The health-related portion of Physical Best, however, does not offer percentile norms. Instead, it offers a *single* performance standard for typically developing students at each age level, 5–18, by gender. Since Physical Best's health-related items do not offer percentile norms, this test's use as a placement tool among persons who have disabilities may be of somewhat limited value (see Chapter Seven, Sampling of Fitness Tests [AAHPERD Physical Best], for further explanation). These tests, particularly where they are norm-referenced, may become a part of the process that determines the degree to which a student with a disability departs from development deemed typical. Overall fitness data can tell the teacher how a student compares with a national average in fitness subtest areas. Teachers can subsequently make decisions and plan instruction around areas of strength and need. Results of such assessments can help determine whether the student with a disability meets entry or exit criteria for placement in adapted physical education.

At middle and high school levels, physical educators may administer tests corresponding to certain curricular units of instruction. For example, the teacher may select a soccer skills test for use at the end of a soccer unit. In a skills test, students are asked to demonstrate proficiencies in specific skills presented during the physical education class. Secondary level physical educators may also administer group fitness tests, and sometimes may administer written tests to assess students' knowledge of physical education concepts.

Today, most physical education curricula are objective-based with clearly defined achievement criteria for each grade level. Objective-based curricula readily lend themselves to ongoing criterion-referenced assessment. In some schools, physical education teachers must report their classes' percentage of mastery on curricular objectives taught during the school year. Objective-based programs with curriculum-imbedded assessment provide a clearly defined system for program evaluation, individualizing instruction, and monitoring pupil progress toward objectives. Objective-based instruction has had tremendous impact on physical education. Curriculum planning, accountability, and curriculum-imbedded assessment are now integral parts of a field in which individualization, heretofore, had seemed to some to be next to impossible.

Regular and adapted physical educators recently have been faced with the challenge of conducting diagnostic tests. Assessment for diagnostic purposes requires that the teacher gather data that helps determine the specific nature of a student's motor difficulties. For example, diagnostic motor testing is utilized to pin-point particular motor development problem areas such as agility or hand-eye coordination. In-depth, diagnostic assessment of motor functioning usually is administered individually. Diagnostic instruments may be formal (e.g., norm-referenced) and/or informal (e.g., criterion-referenced). Formal diagnostic tests often may be administered in one session. Criterion-referenced tests tend to be more time consuming and may require a separate session for each objective area.

Because diagnostic tests usually are administered to students individually, it is difficult for the mainstream physical educator to find time to test such children. In some school districts, adapted physical educators assume responsibility for all movement-related individual assessments.

The content of skills tests administered by physical educators can vary and may include tests of sports skills, fundamental motor skills, or perceptual-motor abilities. Contents of these tests should be directly reflective of skills taught in the physical education curriculum, and skills in the curriculum should be directly reflective of skills needed in community and home-based settings.

Assessment by the Recreation Therapist

To some degree all recreation is therapeutic. The range of activities perceived to be recreational is limited virtually only by the eye of the beholder. While physical education, including adapted physical education, primarily addresses development in the psychomotor domain (i.e., playing tennis, going skiing, engaging in aerobics), recreation encompasses activities which are both motor *and* nonmotor. Recreation may be very active or very sedentary. Depending on any given individual's unique interests and needs, recreation experience can range from sport parachuting (very active) to playing a video game (very sedentary). Any worthwhile activity in which a person might participate during discretionary time can become the focus of leisure assessment. Often there will be potential for overlap between assessments conducted by both APE and TR specialists. In these instances, truly concerned professionals must strive to concentrate less on territorial imperatives and more on what eventually can transpire as participation opportunity offered in the best interest of the person being served.

Knowing the client's developmental history will enable the TR specialist to determine how the client has achieved (including how long it has taken the client to achieve) his or her present status. The TR specialist also needs to become informed of the client's current leisure awareness (i.e., does he or she appreciate, to the extent he or she is capable, the value of meaningful leisure experience, and, if so, is she or he aware of available leisure resources?). Getting to know the client should also focus on assessing what the client perceives to be barriers to his or her engaging in leisure activity. If the client, for whatever reason, cannot address the barriers issue, the TR specialist and/or a significant other, acting on the client's behalf, must do so.

The Joint Commission on Accreditation of Hospitals [JCAH] (1981) has identified what it considers to be essential components of any inquiry whose purpose is to get to know the student/client. According to JCAH, getting to know the client for facilitating therapeutic recreation involves getting to know the client's (1) interests, (2) current skills, (3) aptitudes, (4) talents, (5) needs, (6) life experiences, (7) capabilities, and (8) deficiencies.

Any process in getting to know a client must include assessment of the client's strengths and limitations in relation to what successful participation in a given program will require of the client. For example, will a client with multiple sclerosis be reasonably able to participate in a canoe expedition where there is a necessity to transfer into and out of the canoe, carry a pack, and negotiate rocky portages? Given that the answer is an unqualified "yes," the client likely may participate unabetted.

Given that the answer is a qualified "yes," qualifications need to be addressed to determine if modifications can be made to effect a positive, meaningful canoe expedition experience.

Assessments by Specialists Representing Other Therapies

In recent years, schools have become more interdisciplinary in their approaches to providing opportunities for students who have disabilities. An important manifestation of this trend is that occupational therapists (OTs) and physical therapists (PTs) have undertaken new, contributing roles in public schools. Pursuant to federal mandates, these therapies are provided as related services when determined necessary to facilitate the student's special education program.

When therapists are members of the child study team, portions of motor assessment can be conducted by the OT or PT. Traditionally, OTs and PTs have functioned within a medical model while physical educators have functioned within an educational model. Physical education teachers primarily assess observable, measurable motor skills, while OTs and PTs tend to assess processes underlying movement. For example, the physical educator might assess throwing skill while the physical therapist might assess range of motion that, in part, underlies the ability to throw skillfully. Given yet another example, the OT might assess manipulative abilities that facilitate ball handling which, in turn, affect throwing proficiency. OTs and PTs, like adapted physical educators and recreational therapists, conduct both formal and informal assessments.

Occupational therapists in school settings might administer formal or informal tests to identify a student's functional performance levels in the following areas (Gilfoyle 1981):

1. Gross and fine motor skills
2. Reflex and reaction development
3. Developmental landmarks
4. Sensorimotor functioning
5. Neuromuscular functioning
6. Self-help skills
7. Prevocational skills
8. Social interaction skills

Several assessment areas overlap with adapted physical education, therapeutic recreation, and special education. This sort of overlap of professional responsibilities has been the subject of some controversy. Therapists and educators, however, can work cooperatively to avoid both gaps in assessment and service. Upon receiving and reviewing the referral of a student/client for assessment, it is vital that physical educators and therapists cooperatively plan and decide who will administer each type of assessment. Each professional has unique, relevant information to bring to the team meeting. The interdisciplinary approach to assessment emphasizes sharing, respecting, and learning from each team member's contribution.

In some schools, physical therapists are available to assist in motor assessment. For students who have physical disabilities (e.g., cerebral palsy, muscular dystrophy), motor assessment may be based primarily on a medical model. Evaluation conducted by a physical therapist can provide valuable insights for planning appropriate physical activities. Physical therapists can evaluate tonus, range of motion, posture patterns, and movement patterns. Results of a clinical evaluation of motor functioning by a physical therapist are then combined with information gathered by a physical educator. In cases involving physically disabling conditions when only early diagnostic information is available, a current evaluation by a physical therapist may shed light on present functional capacity and subsequent implications for physical education programming. In addition to identifying physiological (motor), topographical (affected parts of body), and etiological (causative) factors used in classifying physical disabilities, physical therapists can also conduct supplemental evaluations including:

1. Physical status (growth, developmental level, bone age)
2. Posture evaluation
3. Eye-hand behavior patterns (eye dominance, eye movements, fixation, convergence, grasp)
4. Visual status (sensory defects, motor defects)
5. Early reflexes
6. Joint range of motion and strength
7. Motor skill levels (locomotor, head control, trunk control)
8. Motor symptoms (spasticity, athetosis, ataxia, rigidity, tremors)

Although PTs can provide information vital to the physical educator, intervention becomes the point of departure for the two disciplines. The therapist's and educator's challenge is to translate relevant evaluative information into appropriate educational goals and objectives for the individual student/client. Within the context of the educational setting, objectives defined for the student/client must be observable and measurable, and based on the educational model (rather than therapeutic goals within the medical model, which are more appropriately addressed in clinical settings).

References

American Alliance for Health, Physical Education, Recreation, and Dance. *Youth Fitness Test.* Washington, D.C.: The Alliance, 1976.

American Alliance for Health, Physical Education, Recreation, and Dance. *Health Related Fitness Test.* Reston, VA: The Alliance, 1980.

American Alliance for Health, Physical Education, Recreation, and Dance. *Physical Best Test.* Reston, VA: The Alliance, 1988.

Gilfoyle, E. M. *Training: Occupational Therapy Educational Management in Schools.* Washington, D.C.: U.S. Office of Rehabilitative Services, 1981.

Joint Commission on Accreditation of Hospitals. *Consolidated Standards Manual for Child, Adolescent, and Adult Psychiatric, Alcoholism, and Abuse Programs.* Chicago, IL: JCAH, 1981.

Seaman, J. A., and K. P. DePauw. *The New Adapted Physical Education: A Developmental Approach,* 2nd ed. Mountain View, CA: Mayfield, 1989.

CHAPTER 4

Can the Measurement Be Trusted?

Reasons for administering tests (i.e., collecting data) are many and interrelated. The interpretation of data which follows testing (i.e., assessment) serves a variety of essential purposes (see Chapter Two).

The significance of assessment in virtually all aspects of APE and TR cannot be overemphasized. Assessment provides the basis for justifying and evaluating virtually everything we do. Given the pervasive significance of assessment in all facets of APE and TR, it is essential that data providing the very basis for assessment be trustworthy. Always, while data are being collected and analyzed, the question must be asked, "Can the data be trusted?" The answer must be "yes," and until "yes" is forthcoming, any assessment resulting from questionable data must be considered suspect.

More often than not, the answer to "Can the data be trusted?" will be a qualified "yes." It is difficult, if not impossible, to collect data, particularly in practical settings, that are not contaminated or compromised in some way. Often, factors affecting the outcome of testing are not fully within the teacher's/leader's control. For example, the student/client might come to the test with the flu or a headache. There may have been some family stress that morning at home. The temperature and/or humidity might have been elevated during testing. Distractions during testing (e.g., noise from other activity near the test site) could have compromised the person's ability to stay on task. A test administered at the beginning of the day when the person tends to be relatively rested and alert might yield different results from one administered late in the afternoon just before the school bus arrives. Sometimes, even when most or all of the foregoing concerns have been effectively addressed, a test or test item, simply because it is poorly constructed, will yield untrustworthy information.

As APE and TR specialists, we must recognize the necessity for knowing when and when not to have confidence in data that provide bases for making programmatic decisions. Here, an expression from computer science is applicable. The admonition "garbage in, garbage out" speaks graphically to the fact that all tests yield data. When the data are of questionable integrity, but, for whatever reason, are used to make programmatic decisions, of what value are those decisions? One must not simply place faith in a given test, whether it be published and allegedly standardized or teacher-made. Even when we have judged a test satisfactory for a given purpose, we must remain aware of aforementioned factors extrinsic to the test that can affect the trustworthiness of data yielded. When determining trustworthiness of test data, scholarly scrutiny should be the rule, and the following considerations are in order.

Validity

If a test measures what it alleges to measure, that test is said to be *valid.* Among persons new to assessment in general and particularly assessment specific to APE and TR, the concept of validity seems deceptively simple. Perhaps because the concept of validity seems simplistic, concern for validity by both test developers and test users is sometimes inadequate. There are a number of facets to validity. All are important, and the following are cases in point.

Content Validity

All programs have content. Many programs, including those in APE and TR, have embedded within them tests to determine the degree to which the individual has benefited from participation. Both teacher/leader and participant need to know what has been learned as a result of participation. For content validity's sake, tests to determine what a learner has learned must accurately reflect that which the program has endeavored to teach. For example, if a program devotes 40 percent emphasis to fitness development, 40 percent emphasis to skill development, and 20 percent emphasis to related knowledge development, the totality of tests within that program, to have content validity, must have 40 percent of its items addressing fitness, 40 percent of its items addressing skill, and 20 percent of its items addressing related knowledge.

Physical and motor fitness tests, sometimes because of their brevity, can present problems with respect to content validity. Consider that physical and motor fitness consists of 11 items which largely exist mutually exclusively of one another. Let us assume that these items are as follows:

Physical Fitness	**Motor Fitness**
1. Muscular strength	1. Balance
2. Muscular endurance	2. Speed
3. Flexibility	3. Reaction time
4. Cardiovascular endurance	4. Coordination
5. Body composition	5. Agility
	6. Power

Now, assume (as is often the case) that a given test of physical and motor fitness consists of fewer than 11 items. If the above 11 components could be construed to represent the content of fitness, then a fitness test, to have content validity, would have to address performance in each of the 11 performance domains. To satisfy concern for content validity, such a test would require at least 11 items, each of which measured proficiency within each specific, mutually exclusive performance domain. What is one to do when a single fitness test battery does not address every fitness component? One possible solution is to seek out and administer items from a number of technically adequate tests until there is assurance that all components of fitness for which there are concern are covered.

Tests lacking in content validity have potential to yield at least two distinct kinds of misinformation. Such tests are likely either to overestimate or underestimate the person's abilities. For example, let us say that health-related fitness consists of five components including (1) muscular strength, (2) muscular endurance, (3) flexibility, (4) cardiovascular endurance, and (5) body composition. Let us also say that each component receives equal emphasis in the curriculum. Now, a fitness test is given, but the test in question does not measure flexibility to the degree that flexibility is emphasized in the curriculum. If the person's flexibility is very good (e.g., person is an advanced-level Special Olympics gymnastics participant), his or her fitness likely will be underestimated. Why? Because the test does not recognize the person's flexibility to the degree that it is valued in the curriculum. If the person's flexibility is poor, his or her fitness likely will be overestimated. Why? Again, because the test is not sensitive to the individual's flexibility fitness which the curriculum values.

Concern for a test's content validity is essential when the test is used to determine the appropriateness of placing a given participant in an existing program. When a test administered prior to program placement has content validity (i.e., reflects what the program in question will teach), those interpreting test results can accurately determine whether the program in question is appropriate for a given individual.

Finally, concern for test content validity is essential when determining present achievement levels as a prerequisite to developing a student's/client's individualized education or therapy program. A test with content validity, in this instance, is sensitive to what needs to be learned, and thereby reveals what learning needs to take place. Subsequently, an individualized program can be fashioned, emphasizing the individual's unique, test-identified learning needs. Assessment from this perspective molds programs to fit individuals rather than individuals to fit programs. This perspective, which respects the uniqueness of the individual, reflects the very essence of truly individualized instruction.

Construct Validity

A test item is said to have construct validity if performance on the item in question is truly representative of the performance domain it alleges to represent. Take, for example, the motor performance domain agility. Characteristically, the shuttle run historically has been an accepted agility measure. Using the shuttle run as an example, concern for construct validity begs the question, "Does the shuttle run truly measure agility?" The answer to this question helps determine whether, in fact, the item actually does measure agility. In certain instances, the aforementioned agility run has been found to be lacking in construct validity. For example, among children with mental retardation, agility run results have been shown to correlate significantly with mental age (Speakman, 1977). The effect is that, among persons with mental retardation, higher mental age is statistically significantly correlated with faster agility run times. Agility runs among persons with mental retardation therefore do not have construct validity, because among such persons, an agility run is not truly measuring agility. In this case, the agility run may be little more than a sloppy measure of mental age.

Construct validity is questionable any time a test item measures more than one proficiency. In such instances, the tester often cannot clearly ascertain to what degree each proficiency is contributing to a single score. For example, a score in the 50-yard dash, allegedly a measure of speed, is confounded by the effects of additional performance components of reaction time and power. Does a slow 50-yard dash time indicate poor speed, slow reaction time, inadequate power, or some combination of the three (see Figure 4.1)? In this instance, what valid interpretation can a teacher make from such data? One solution might be to specify a flying start, thereby minimizing contributions of reaction time and explosive strength to the student's elapsed time. Remember, however, that whenever norms are used, test items must be administered exactly as specified in the test manual. Otherwise said norms would not be valid. If the teacher/ leader, out of concern for construct validity, were to incorporate the flying start 50-yard dash as an alternative to the traditional 50-yard dash, he or she would either have to go in search of norms for that specific measure, or could develop local norms after having gathered a sufficient quantity of flying start 50-yard dash data.

Figure 4.2 reveals yet another often used test item, this one allegedly measuring throwing skill, wherein construct validity is questionable. The item relies on a series of concentric rectangles, rather than concentric circles, to assess throwing accuracy. A construct validity problem arises, because accuracy deviations, resulting in ball contacts at 3 or 9 o'clock on the rectangular target are more severely penalized than deviations in the 12 and 6 o'clock directions. The tester must ask if this specific procedure has been prescribed for some specific reason

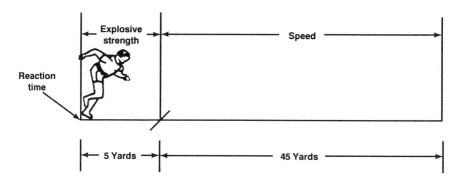

FIGURE 4.1 Does the 50-yard dash measure speed alone, or is speed measurement complicated by inclusion of related proficiencies such as reaction time and explosive strength?

or if the test developer erred with respect to construct validity in the attempt to measure accuracy.

A construct validity problem seems apparent in at least one item appearing in a motor proficiency battery often used for placement purposes in APE. This item, from the Bruininks-Oseretsky Test of Motor Proficiency (Bruininks, 1978) is called Running Speed and Agility. The construct validity dilemma associated with this item rests in the fact that the item, as indicated by its name, is measuring two components of performance. Yet, the item yields only one score. How can one know for certain how much of the single score that combines speed and agility is representative of speed and how much is representative of agility? The answer simply is that one cannot objectively make that determination. A good test item, to facilitate meaningful interpretation of the item's score, must measure one behavior only.

The foregoing are examples of test items that raise construct validity questions. This delineation of examples is far from exhaustive. These examples are provided for the primary purpose of getting the reader to consider the far reaching significance of construct validity when judging the worth of entire tests and specific test items.

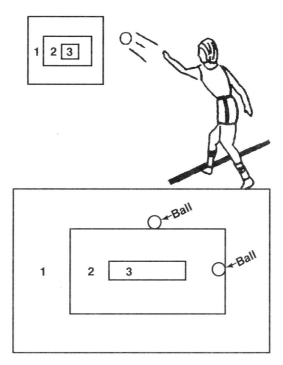

FIGURE 4.2 Item testing throwing accuracy, Township of Ocean Physical Fitness Test (Vodola, 1976). Both balls are equidistant from the target center, yet one throw is awarded two points (3 o'clock) and the other is awarded one point (1 o'clock).

Concurrent Validity

When two test batteries yield essentially the same result, those tests are said to have concurrent validity. At times, the APE or TR specialist may want to switch from one test to another. Perhaps motivation for such a switch rests in the belief that a different, perhaps newer, test may be more easily administrable. First, there must be the assumption that the tester is satisfied with the validity of the old test. If results of the new test yield results essentially equal to those of the old test, the tester may, with confidence, switch to the new test. Concurrent validity between tests helps ensure that essentially the same information provided by the old test can now be provided by the new test. Correlation techniques (e.g., correlating results of test A with test B) typically provide the basis for making concurrent validity determinations.

Concern for concurrent validity (in this case, a first cousin to content validity) should also arise when the short form of a test is given for purposes of determining whether the test's long form should subsequently be administered. Short forms of tests typically are used in screening settings. They serve to identify persons for whom further evaluation is indicated. If a test's short form score does not correlate at least to some degree with that of its long form (because the respective tests' contents differ), there can be little objective basis for deciding who among those tested might warrant further observation.

Factors Influencing Validity

A person's disposition at test time can affect validity. For example, a child with juvenile rheumatoid arthritis often has "good" days and "bad" days. During times when the disease is particularly active, the child, due to discomfort, moodiness and distractions resulting from discomfort, or lack of sleep, may not perform on a test in a manner that truly reflects her or his best.

The tester's disposition at test time can affect validity. This may be particularly true when scores assigned to the person's performance are the product of the tester's subjective judgment.

Some children's test performances may be affected by medications being taken at test time. For example, drowsiness can be one side effect of some medications prescribed to control seizures. Yet another example is the person with type I (insulin dependent) diabetes who at test time may be experiencing a blood sugar level outside normal parameters. In this case, the person, either hyperglycemic or hypoglycemic, may exhibit both motor and mental functions not reflective of his or her best. Likewise, changes in medications can affect test performance either because a new medication's dosage is still being adjusted, or because a medication taken at posttest time might be different than that taken at pretest time. Finally, the person may have failed to take prescribed medication, and this lack of compliance could manifest itself in altered performance.

Some tests rely on competition to evoke best responses. For example, agility runs and dashes often find two or more persons, side-by-side, striving to outdo the other to achieve the best score. Some children and adults, for numerous reasons, may not relate particularly well to competition. Where competition does precipitate a better test score, the person not relating to competition is at a disadvantage. One obvious consequence of assessment resulting from reliance on a less-than-best test score is diminished expectations on the part of the assessor.

Test standardization procedures must be strictly adhered to in *all* cases. For example, if a test item calls only for three trials, the tester must not offer the person four trials in hope of achieving a better result. If the test item calls for use of a tennis ball, the tester must not substitute a playground ball. Unless standardization procedures are followed with utmost scrutiny, the person's performance will not be equitably comparable to norms or performance criteria provided by the test.

Some persons with mental disabilities may not clearly understand the concept of "do your best." Among those who, indeed, understand this concept, there may exist a discrepancy between teacher/leader and student/client regarding the importance of doing one's best. The person being tested simply may not share the tester's enthusiasm for putting forth a best effort. This situation may arise particularly when doing one's best results in self-inflicted discomfort (e.g., a 1½ mile endurance run).

Many persons with limited abilities relative to proficiencies tested will exhibit attention spans not compatible with completing an entire test in one session. In such instances, both mental and physical fatigue can be factors. The tester must be sensitive to the person's attention span at test time, since results on items nearer the end of the test may not be as indicative of best performances as those from the beginning. Within limitations prescribed by any given test's administration procedures, the tester may need to rely on a variety of ways to attract and maintain the person's interest. When reasonable means to maintain the person's interest have failed, the tester is advised to abandon further testing for the time being.

When determining the appropriateness of a given test for any given individual, the tester must be aware of the population for which the test was intended. For example, when a student being tested is blind, it is appropriate to consider whether students who also are blind were included in the normative group to which this particular student is being compared. In yet another instance, should persons with severe mental retardation ever be subjected to norms developed for persons with moderate mental retardation? Were persons from your student's/client's locale included in the development of norms? Since regional differences in performance sometimes affect norms, norms should be drawn from large, representative samples of peers.

Generally, when norms are applied to a given student/client, that student/client should be compared with peers. Perhaps the most notable exception to this rule is when a person with a disability is being tested to determine how far his or her present achievement level departs from achievement deemed typical. At this point, it is appropriate, with caution, to compare the score of a person with a disability to norms derived from the typically developing population.

When making this comparison it is critical that a particular test item not discriminate unfairly on the basis of disability. The aforementioned agility run among persons with mental retardation offers a case in point (see **Construct Validity,** this chapter). Any test item, to be valid, must measure the behavioral component it purports to measure. It must not measure the degree to which disability impedes performance with respect to that component. Simply stated, an agility run should measure agility, not mental retardation.

Sometimes, test developers have been forced to rely on less than optimum sample sizes when compiling norms. This is particularly true when norms are developed for persons with disabilities. One case in point is Project UNIQUE (Winnick and Short, 1985) where, despite the effort to secure adequate sample sizes, norm group sizes for a given age and gender sometimes did not exceed 20.

Whenever possible, the tester should note the number of persons tested during norm development to determine the representativeness of norms. When the number in a normative group is relatively small from one age group to another for any given test item, the examiner may note a phenomenon known as *spiking norms*. Figure 4.3, an excerpt from the *Motor Fitness Testing Manual for the Moderately Mentally Retarded* (AAHPERD, 1976), offers an example of spiking norms resulting from inadequate sample size.

Another concern when applying norms is that norms, to be useful, must discriminate among different levels of proficiency. If norms are not challenging and if everyone exceeds the 90th percentile, or if norms are so challenging that no one exceeds the 10th percentile, what basis does the teacher/leader have for determining relative abilities? Norms applied should be sensitive to varied abilities of persons within the group. Further, when development of the person being tested is substantially delayed, the tester may need to consider a test developed for younger populations. For example, the Battelle Developmental Inventory (Newborg, Stock, and Whek, 1984) is normed for persons ages 0–8. If a 15-year-old is functioning motorically at approximately a 7-year level, the motor development sector of the Battelle might be appropriate for this person.

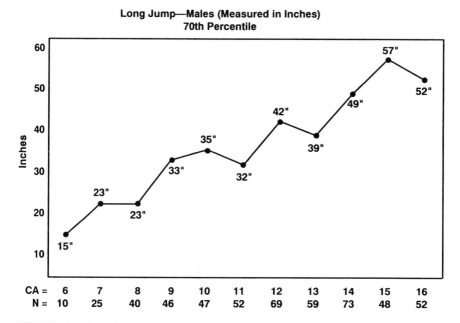

FIGURE 4.3 Example of spiking norms (*Motor Fitness Testing Manual for the Moderately Mentally Retarded*, AAHPERD, 1976). (CA = chronological age; N = number in sample)

Some persons, particularly children still in the process of acquiring language, may have vocabularies that limit their abilities to process verbal information. A child instructed to throw the ball as *fast* as she or he can may understand clearly. Yet, if that same child is instructed to throw the ball as *hard* as she or he can, she or he may not understand the task at all. When the student's/client's vocabulary is limited, the tester should attempt to identify key words or terms to communicate the behavior desired. In this way, key words are not obscured by those less important. An example of this technique is found in *I CAN* assessment procedures wherein specific action words are identified and recommended for use by the test developer (Kelly and Wessel, 1990).

In considering the person's language development level, the APE and TR specialist should be aware of both expressive and receptive language abilities. Expressive language refers to language the person speaks. Receptive language refers to language the person comprehends. Among persons with special needs who have language delays, receptive language development often exceeds expressive language development. Further, the tester may encounter a person for whom English is a second language. Concern for validity then turns to ensuring that the test is administered in the person's native tongue.

For some children with hearing impairments, signing and finger spelling are the preferred modes of communication. Signs and finger spellings must then become the communications mode through which test instructions are provided. When hard-of-hearing persons do rely in part or full on speech, the examiner, when speaking, must always face the student. The examiner's speech patterns should not be altered (i.e., do not overpronounce words), and, when possible, the student's back should be toward the sun or any bright lights. Note also that moustaches or beards that obscure the speaker's lips are particularly problematic for persons who rely on speech reading for communication.

In test-retest or pretest-posttest situations, the teacher/leader must be certain that test conditions during the second administration are identical to those during the first administration. Is the time of day similar? Is the time of week similar? Are weather conditions similar? If the child uses a brace or assistive device for ambulation, was such a device (even more specifically, the same device) used during the first test? Is a wheelchair user using the same or at least the same quality chair as during the first test? Has wheelchair maintenance improved or deteriorated during the ensuing time? Is the same person administering the test? The foregoing are but a few examples of the many factors that can influence results in test/retest or pretest/posttest situations. Unless such factors are considered in such situations, results may be wholly or partially invalid.

All of the above represent only a few of the factors that can affect validity in any APE or TR testing situation. The foregoing factors affecting validity should not be perceived as exhaustive. Rather, they are offered to heighten sensitivity to phenomena that can affect validity, and hence the degree to which the measurement can be trusted.

Reliability

Reliability addresses concern for consistency. A test is deemed reliable if repeated measures, under substantially similar conditions, yield substantially similar results.

For example, a ruler is deemed a reliable measure of a line's length if the same ruler is used when length is recorded during successive trials. In measuring human performance, however, one seldom expects or achieves such precision. It should suffice that the tester be satisfied when an observed proficiency is representative of the person's true ability.

When administering a test item requiring more than one trial (i.e., add the total of three trials or score the best of three trials), one need observe consistency of the student's performances. Consistency tends to reveal reliability. The tester should always be suspect of scores when the quality of performances across trials seems erratic.

When administering items requiring that the person demonstrate stamina, relatively few trials (perhaps only one) tend to yield greatest reliability. For example, were one to execute as many pull-ups as possible in three successive trials, the first trial, due to progressive fatigue, likely would yield the most reliable score. On the other hand, with items measuring skill (e.g., throwing accuracy), increased successive trials would likely yield the most accurate data.

One should not be bound by any predesignated number of trials when one makes up one's own test. Here, the teacher/leader, as test developer, can determine how many trials per item will yield the most reliable scores. When experimenting with a test item for reliability purposes, the teacher/leader must address two concerns regarding optimum numbers of trials. First, there should be sufficient trials to yield consistent scores. Second, the number of trials should be limited to as few as possible (without compromising reliability) so that administration of the test item does not measure the learning effect and is time-effective.

Many factors affecting validity also affect reliability. For example, any alteration in a person's medication prescription or medication schedule could influence performance. If a person took her or his medication yesterday and were tested yesterday, results might be different than if the person were tested today, but had forgotten to take the medication before coming to the program this morning. Reliability, in this example, would be suspect, because the person's scores yesterday and today quite likely might be different. Here, consistency across trials would be suspect.

For reliability's sake, objectivity in scoring tends to facilitate reliability. For example, the number of cards sorted in 30 seconds is quite objectively measurable. If one were to count the number of cards sorted for a given trial, and then recount the number of cards, one would most likely come up with the same number. On the other hand, objectivity would be more questionable when counting the number of correct steps in a beam walking test, given that the success criterion is that one step be no further than 1 inch (toe-to-heel) from the next step. Actually, two reliability questions need to be raised at this juncture: (1) how objectively scorable is the item, and (2) given that the item is objectively scorable, will that score be repeatable across trials?

Items that yield *quantifiable* scores (i.e., numbers of pull-ups, pulse, numbers of cards sorted, numbers of items placed in a container) tend to be relatively more reliable than items yielding rating scale scores (i.e., always, sometimes, never). Assignment of rating scale scores tends to be more dependent on the subjective (as opposed to objective) judgment of the rater. Whenever rating scales provide the basis for gathering data, concern for reliability dictates that rating criteria be stated as objectively as possible.

Objectivity

Objectivity is an important aspect of reliability. It addresses the degree to which two or more scorers, rating the same performance, assign to that performance identical, or at least reasonably identical, scores. Where reliability addresses scoring consistency across trials, objectivity addresses scoring consistency across raters. For example, were two raters to read a person's weight as measured by a digital scale, each likely would record the same score. Here, objectivity would be optimal. The same would be true if two raters simultaneously were to count the number of sit-ups executed by a student. As with reliability, the more objectively measurable the item, the greater will be the objectivity coefficient between or among raters.

Often, wholly objectively measurable data simply cannot be derived from observing a given performance or behavior. For example, judging the routines of Special Olympics floor exercise contestants invites subjectivity. If one has ever witnessed inconsistencies among raters scoring the same performance (e.g., as in gymnastics, diving, figure skating), one has witnessed a problem in objectivity.

One significant factor affecting the results' objectivity, whether they be of the stopwatch (objective) or rating scale (subjective) type, is rapport between examiner and student/client. Typically, the better the rapport, the better the score. For whatever reason, gender and age of the student versus gender and age of the examiner may influence the person's performance. Among some students/clients, one examiner's demeanor may be more reassuring (or threatening) than that of another. Results can be affected by the presence of others at test time, and, further, by whether those present are asserting positive, neutral, or negative influence. When others are in attendance, who the others are becomes important. Parents, siblings, peers, friends, and authority figures all can have differing influences on the person's performance. When such influences are present during some test times but not during others and when more than one examiner assigns scores, both reliability and objectivity of scores should be questioned.

Objectivity is of particular significance whenever one person's test results are to be interpreted by another person. If the person interpreting the data might have assigned scores different from those with whom he or she is working, then an individualized program based on those scores would probably take on a different emphasis. These circumstances render test objectivity questionable, and thus render validity questionable. Objectivity (also known as interrater reliability) can be calculated when more than one person observes a student's/client's scores by calculating **percent of agreement:**

$$\frac{\text{Agreements}}{\text{Agreements + Disagreements}} \times 100 = \% \text{ Agreement}$$

The assessment is considered adequate if the interrater reliability is at least 80 percent.

Relationship Between Validity and Reliability

Reliability and validity are interrelated, because one cannot achieve validity without first having achieved reliability. A reliable measurement does not automatically guarantee a valid measurement. For example, a scale might consistently (i.e., reliably) weigh someone at 125 pounds. However, the scale may not have been calibrated carefully, and may be weighing everyone 5 pounds heavy. Here, weight is being reliably measured, but the measures, due to inaccurate scale calibration, are simply not valid. In yet another example, if a tester were to measure balance by repeated foot placements on a 4-inch-wide stripe painted on the floor, a quantifiable score would result. If more than one performance yielded consistent scores, the tester might rightly suspect those scores to be reliable. Given these data, students/clients could be ranked according to balance beam ability. Now, assume that the same task were repeated, only the stripe is now replaced by a 4-inch-wide beam placed 2 feet above the ground. If rankings on the elevated beam are different, could both items have measured the same ability (i.e., balance)? While performance on the relatively less threatening stripe measured balance, performance on the relatively more threatening elevated beam might have measured courage in addition to balance. Both items may have yielded reliable information, but interpreting the latter data in terms of balance would render the item's validity suspect. An item, even though reliable, must not therefore be considered automatically valid.

When Tests Are Less than Perfect

No test is perfect, and no testing environment is ever completely adequate. At best, the teacher/leader must strive to achieve testing conditions that fall somewhere between less than perfect and more than adequate. Achievement of this goal is facilitated when the teacher assumes the role of both detective and scholar. Recognizing that some tests are technically inadequate and that testing environments are sometimes not conducive to eliciting best responses, the teacher is compelled to rely on her or his best professional judgment when interpreting test results. By recognizing as many factors as possible that limit data trustworthiness, we take a critical initial step toward minimizing the potential negative impact that such factors will have on important assessment functions.

References

American Alliance for Health, Physical Education, Recreation, and Dance. *Motor Fitness Testing Manual for the Moderately Mentally Retarded.* Washington, D.C.: The Alliance, 1976.

Bruininks, R.H. *Bruininks-Oseretsky Test of Motor Proficiency.* Circle Pines, MN: American Guidance Service, 1978.

Kelly, L., and J.A. Wessel. *I CAN: Primary Skills.* Austin, TX: Pro-Ed, 1990.

Newborg, J., J.R. Stock, and L.Whek. *Battelle Developmental Inventory.* Allen, TX: 1984.

Speakman, H.G.B. "A Motor Fitness Test Suitable for Trainable Mentally Retarded Children." *Arkansas Journal for Health, Physical Education, and Recreation,* 12:8–10, 1977.

Vodola, T. *Project Active Maximodel: Nine Training Manuals.* Oakhurst, NJ: Project Active, 1976.

Winnick, J.P., and F.X. Short. *Physical Fitness Testing of the Disabled: Project UNIQUE.* Champaign, IL: Human Kinetics, 1985.

CHAPTER 5

Test Selection and Administration Insights

A valid and reliable assessment process considers three factors that influence performance: (1) task demands, (2) medical history and characteristics of the individual, and (3) environmental factors inherent in the assessment process and setting. Assessment is not merely the administration of a test, but the entire process of gathering information in an ecological approach (Davis and Burton, 1991). A major part of a comprehensive assessment process involves gathering information apart from formal and informal testing procedures. Parent and teacher observations of movement or behaviors are important sources of assessment information that may prove useful in determining the individual's functional capabilities. Assessment is a process of gathering, evaluating, interpreting, and appraising information about an individual's performance.

Ways to Gather Information

The gathering of information about physical and motor performance can be generated from a variety of settings or situations. In educational or clinical settings, formal and informal tests are tools for gathering information required to develop program plans. To determine which assessment instrument is appropriate, the purpose of the assessment should be considered. Test selection should be undertaken with extreme care to satisfy validity and reliability standards as well as to be appropriate for (1) screening, (2) placement, (3) instructional planning, (4) functional skill development, and (5) reviewing progress to determine which formal and informal test procedures are best.

Some of the specific administration concerns that should be considered in selecting a test instrument include:

1. Economical in terms of time and equipment
2. Appropriate to unique characteristics, including physical, intellectual, and emotional development

3. Comprehensive in providing essential information to meet the purposes of the test (e.g., screening, placement, progress review, program planning)
4. Familiarity with test and procedures
5. Ensure group testing if appropriate
6. Be easy to set up or move (appropriate in field-based settings)
7. Provide appropriate information (e.g., norms or useful scores)
8. Be specific to program planning or evaluation

Test Characteristics

Baumgartner and Jackson (1995) reported that certain characteristics are essential to develop and select appropriate evaluation instruments. These characteristics should include the ecological approach and be concerned with the individuals tested, the procedure for administration, the objectives and attributes of the test, and the acceptability in making generalizations about the test scores. Several characteristics recommended by Baumgartner and Jackson (1995) include:

1. *Reliability, Objectivity, Validity*—These are the most important characteristics of a test. Test-retest reliability above .85, objectivity above .85, validity above .80 for fitness tests, and above .70 for spot skill tests, although the validity coefficients may be dependent on the criterion selected.
2. *Discrimination*—The ability to differentiate among ability groups is critical with persons with disabilities. Since persons with disabilities vary immensely in functional capabilities, the test must have a distribution of scores with no zero or perfect scores.
3. *Specificity*—The instrument utilized should be task specific. While some measures may combine several attributes, others may test a single factor. For persons with disabilities, determining functional skill level may require several attributes to adequately assess functional capabilities.
4. *Appropriateness*—Since the search for a single measurement item or test for persons with disabilities does not exist, performance must be based on age, maturation, severity level, and cognitive ability in selecting an instrument. Likewise, comparing performances of children or peers without disabilities may not be appropriate if the scores generated do not give an adequate picture of their capabilities.
5. *Individuality*—According to Baumgartner and Jackson (1995), test scores should not be affected by another's performance. In addition, wide variations in some disabilities and capabilities will vary according to individuals and effects of intervention.
6. *Safety*—Safety is a factor in all testing and should be adhered to for persons with disabilities. Test procedures should not overtax weakened muscle groups or put an individual in a situation where symptoms may be exacerbated.
7. *Motivation*—One of the most difficult tasks in assessment is motivating participants to perform to their capabilities. Some individuals may

require prompting and urging to complete the test. In contrast, the results of some assessments hopefully will encourage other individuals to continue their activity and improvement. Finally, some days or settings may not be conducive to good results and more data points should be utilized.

Formal Tests

Frequently, the terms test, measurement, and evaluation are used interchangeably. In this text, formal testing is considered to be the narrowest concept, meaning the presentation of a standard set of items that require a response. As a result of an individual's movement responses to a given series of formal motor test items, we obtain a measure, that is, a numerical value, of a motor characteristic of that individual.

In the educational or clinical context, the evaluator directs the individual to execute a specific task or motor skill. Directions to the individual must follow a standard procedure given in the administration guidelines of the test manual. When the individual executes the desired motor skill, the evaluator assigns a score to the individual's performance according to the test's standardized scoring procedure.

To ensure validity and reliability, the evaluator must be thoroughly familiar with the test and learn standardized procedures for administering the test. When administering a formal test, directions are usually verbal and may involve some demonstration. For individuals who may have difficulty understanding or attending to the directions, the evaluator may decide to rephrase the directions. Although this may be permissible, the evaluator should not indiscriminately alter the test procedures and should adhere to the test manual guidelines regarding the presentation and possible alteration of verbal or visual directions.

In addition, formal tests usually have other standard procedures that must be followed in order to preserve standardized conditions. Besides administering the test, the tester must also establish the testing environment, introduce the individual to the testing situation, use appropriate test equipment, and observe performance according to the test's standardized procedures. Each procedure should be followed with rigorous guidelines to ensure generalizability of results to others.

Test Environment

When establishing the test environment, a simple checklist can be used to rate the adequacy of the testing room, space, and equipment (see Table 5.1). The appropriate test environment is essential for proper administration of the test. Many responses may require adequate space for throwing, running, jumping, or performing floor exercises. To generate information required for appropriate placement and program planning, a consistent environment is essential for comparing and assessing the individual's capabilities. Likewise, the test environment should closely parallel the learning environment or functional tasks the individual will ultimately perform.

TABLE 5.1 Test Environment Checklist

		Environment Checklist		
Room	Test Requirement	Optimal	Adequate	Poor
Ceiling height				
Distance				
Lighting				
Temperature/ventilation				
Noise level				
Freedom from distractions				
Breakable items				
Windows				
Floor surface				
Safety				
Unnecessary furniture				

Preparing the Subject

An important consideration in preparation is to introduce the subjects to the testing situation including equipment, time of day, and physical and psychological needs. If equipment is used, adequate experimentation or trials should be implemented to ensure understanding of the task. Also, test procedures should be checked to guarantee that practice opportunities are appropriate and do not violate the standardized procedures of the test. For example, practicing items on tests of flexibility or muscle strength would be helpful for the individual to understand test procedures without giving the individual an unfair advantage. The administration of a formal test is usually scheduled in cooperation with other teachers or parents.

Physical needs, such as hunger, thirst, or a visitation to the restroom, should be considered prior to the test. If a disability requires an orthopedic, supportive, or other device, the tester must consider the option of testing without such devices. For example, if an individual wears leg braces, glasses, a hearing aid, or uses a communication board, should he or she be tested with such devices? The tester must consider the purpose of the assessment and how that information will relate to the individual's education plan. If the purpose is to evaluate current functioning in a generalized situation, then devices should be kept in place to maximize validity. In contrast, if the intent is to determine strength without leg braces, the most naturalistic setting will provide the best data. Likewise, the effects of medication should be considered prior to administration of medication. Sufficient time is needed to ensure that the effects of medications are appropriate to generalize test results.

Establishing familiarization with the test will aid in generating appropriate cooperation and results that provide useful information about the individual's functional ability. Prior information, including the following, will be useful in preparing an individual for testing and establishing a comfortable test environment:

1. Behaviors that may interfere with the test
2. Special reinforcement methods that may aid in maintaining attention to test procedures
3. Ways to motivate or prompt the individual
4. Successful methods of communicating directions
5. Strategies to facilitate compliance
6. Attention span and/or level of fatigue
7. Impact of medications on performance

Preparation of the Tester

The tester should prepare to administer the test based on knowledge of the individual, testing situation, and task required. Preparation of subjects prior to testing, or practicing on test items if allowable, can shorten the testing session and allow for a warmup or review. This also allows the individual to become comfortable with the testing environment or instrumentation while the tester gathers information on the style of communication (e.g., monosyllabic, voluble) best for following directions or understanding instructions. A review of the test may be required to eliminate anxiety about the procedure. For example, in some situations individuals with mental retardation were allowed to observe the tester placing a manual muscle tester on their arm and showing the reading generated (Horvat, Croce, and Roswal, 1993). Further, Fernhall and Tymeson (1987) prepared subjects with mental retardation for cardiovascular testing and emphasized (1) laboratory familiarization, (2) ample training time, (3) safety procedures to eliminate falling or fear of falling, (4) adapting the test protocol to the population, and (5) providing a conducive environment of contribution by the participants. In another setting, children become frightened of skinfold calipers because they associate these devices with getting shots. A stated purpose such as "we're going to see how strong you are" denotes a sense of work and may affect the effort displayed as opposed to "we're going to play some games." In contrast, the term "test" should be used cautiously, since individuals may associate unpleasant past experiences or test failures with anxiety or negative connotations. Finally, an explanation of what will transpire with the test should occur prior to or during the testing. For example, Horvat et al. (1993) allowed subjects with mental retardation to practice with the hand-held dynamometer and encouraged them to visualize their efforts prior to formal testing.

Formal tests usually include a set of specific instructions prior to test administration. At times, the individual's functional capabilities may require variations within the context of the test instructions in a language appropriate for the age and ability level. Pretest instructions should include information about the test's length, types of test activities, an indication of test difficulty, whether the tester will be able to help, and an indication of whether some items will be timed. If allowable, some motivation and encouragement should be given to ensure best efforts. If individuals attempt the task halfheartedly it may be appropriate within test standardization to allow another trial or reschedule the test. Also, individuals should indicate if they are becoming uncomfortable or fatigued about any of the test items. Many of the initial studies utilizing hand-held dynamometry with children and individuals with mental retardation indicated that placement of the dynamometer in various positions was uncomfortable and sometimes painful (Horvat, McManis, and Seagraves, 1992; Horvat et al., 1993). The tester should continue careful observation to determine if the individual can perform a task or whether motivation, fatigue, or a short attention span is interfering with performance.

Administration of a Formal Test

When administering a formal test, the test manual guidelines for administering and scoring should be followed, or standardized conditions of the test will be violated. The tester should consult the test manual and vigorously adhere to test standardization on directions, questions, and prompts during the test. Although questioning and encouragement may be permissible when administering formal tests, the tester should never teach the individual, while testing, to achieve the desired response. This would invalidate the response, because each test item was designed and normed on individuals who did not receive coaching.

Recording Responses

Manuals for formal tests include directions for recording responses. Usually a formal test has a recording format or record form. Once the form is completed, the test record is known as the test protocol and constitutes the original record of responses during a formal test. In most instances, the protocol is hidden during the test, since observation of errors may affect the remaining performances in the test.

Most assessments require that the tester observe the performance and score the response simultaneously. Since following scoring guidelines accurately is essential, the demand for instant decisions requires knowledge of testing procedures and scoring quickly and accurately. A thorough study of the recording process and focus on specific criterion to be observed allows for more accurate decisions. For example, a test of muscle strength would always contain a specific criteria that must be met before the repetition is counted, and scoring should remain consistent from trial to trial. Likewise, in a motor assessment such as the Peabody Developmental Motor Scale, criterion for scoring is written into each behavior response, necessitating a valid judgment of the selected criteria if the reliability of the instrument is to be duplicated across testers or settings (Schmidt, Westcott, and Crowe, 1993).

Most formal test forms also provide a space to record informal observations about the test behavior, effort, compliance, or unique characteristics of the individual.

This information may be useful in evaluating the success of the test situation and in further evaluating possible problems such as orthopedic, vision, or hearing difficulties.

Informal Tests

In instructional, home-based, recreational, and clinical settings, the use of informal test procedures can be used to gather information about an individual's functional capabilities in natural environments. In contrast to formal tests, informal test processes generally focus on performance in relation to the demands of the environment. Informal assessment allows the tester to collect information regarding performance from natural settings that may be conducive to developing the formal program plan. These assessment procedures compliment results from formal tests and generate more specific functional information that is essential for program planning. For example, a formal test may indicate that locomotor patterns are deficient. By itself, this information does not allow the teacher to develop a remediation strategy. However, an informal assessment may identify that the individual possesses insufficient muscular strength needed to walk or jump. Obviously, the program plan would then reflect a combination of activities to develop strength, balance, and the specific motor pattern. For some individuals with physical, emotional, intellectual, or sensory impairments, many formal tests may not be available or may not provide the required information to develop an instructional plan. Informal tests may constitute the only appropriate means of assessment in making instructional decisions. They can also provide information for initial screening and assist in making placement decisions for persons with disabilities who cannot be assessed by traditional tests.

Advantages and Disadvantages of Informal Tests

Various informal tests, including naturalistic observation, checklists, task analyses, inventories, rating scales, interviews, and questionnaires are available commercially, or can be designed to meet adequate standards of reliability and validity. A major advantage of informal assessment procedures is the relevance to teaching and program planning. Included in Table 5.2 are various types of informal tests that can be used to formulate program plans and assess performance.

Selecting Informal Tests

Several considerations should be observed when selecting an informal test. First, will the test generate appropriate information (e.g., screening, progress review)? Second, is the test effective in considering efficiency, time of administration, and design? Third, is the test sensitive to developing information regarding program planning? Fourth, what is test quality, and does it adhere to stringent procedures of validity and reliability? In contrast to formal test procedures that ensure a reasonable degree of technical accuracy in terms of reliability and validity, little information is available about the quality of informal tests. Most commercial informal skill tests are not standardized, and few contain validity and reliability information.

TABLE 5.2 Informal Tests and Program Planning

Assessment	Data Generated	Program Planning
Observation	Quantify responses in a naturalistic setting	Determine functional capabilities and effect of intervention
Checklists	Determine sequences necessary for task completion	Determine level of functioning and task achievement
Criterion-referenced tests	Measure performance in comparison to specified criteria	Determine functional capabilities and progress on designated tasks
Task analysis	Measure component parts or subskills of a task or objective	Evaluate performance on stated goals and objectives
Rating scales	Rank performance instead of precise indicator	Estimation of performance
Questionnaire	Accumulation of medical, family or development history	Determination of functional status and effects of disability, medication

From "Ecological Task Analysis: Translating Movement Behavior Theory into Practice" by Davis, W. E., and A. W. Burton, *Adapted Physical Activity Quarterly*, (Vol. 8, No. 2), 162. Copyright 1991 by Human Kinetics Publishers. Reprinted by permission.

When informal tests are designed there can be no assurance about the quality of the procedures if the technical adequacy is not known.

When selecting informal tests, content validity and reliability should be sufficient to guarantee quality results. Content validity can be determined by examining the appropriateness of test items for the content to be evaluated, the range of behaviors, tasks or performances included in the assessment, and the ways in which the items assess the content.

Reliability is also crucial when selecting informal motor tests. Many informal assessments of performance require that someone observe, rate, and/or score the individual's performance. Testers must be relatively confident that their ratings are accurate, as well as being consistent so evaluators would obtain the same results if identical procedures were used. It is recommended that testers estimate the interrater reliability of the informal tests by calculating the percent of agreement as described in Chapter Four.

Observation

Observation of performance provides the most common basis for referral. However, when a potential motor or functional problem is noted, more systematic observation methods may be appropriate. Informal observations can provide information about endurance, strength, locomotor patterns, agility, social interaction, play, or behavior in educational or home-based settings. Such observations can generate usable information in many naturalistic settings that cannot be obtained from other assessment procedures. For example, a teacher may be concerned about the manner in which children interact with others during large-group play activities in the gymnasium. Since the behavior is difficult to assess with a standardized test, observation can be an informal procedure to specify, record, and analyze the behavior as it occurs in the natural setting. The number of appropriate or inappropriate social interactions can then be recorded in the play setting. Observation can be used in continuous recording where all behaviors are observed during a specified time period or be specific to a designated behavior used.

Continuous observation is implemented by recording events during a specified time period to ascertain the situational factors and interactions that may produce specific behaviors. Although effective, continuous recording is time consuming and difficult to execute since watching and writing are performed simultaneously, unless the information is dictated into a cassette or the session is videotaped.

In contrast, specific behavior observations can be conducted to observe a designated behavior or performance during the instructional or play setting. For example, if swimming behavior was to be observed, it is essential to determine a way to accurately measure the desired response. It may be necessary to determine if the behavior is present, such as putting the face into the water or the number of times a behavior occurs. Likewise, it may be appropriate to know the frequency and/or number of attempts to initiate the swimming behavior. The number of specified criteria can then be counted and later used only to count implemented tasks rather than attempts.

Criterion-Referenced Tests and Task Analysis

Criterion-referenced tests (CRTs) are another form of informal assessment. They compare an individual's performance to some criterion rather than to the performance of others as in formal norm-referenced tests. Criterion-referenced tests are usually curriculum based and used to compare skills inherent in the curriculum to the individuals performance (King and Aufsesser, 1988).

Task Analysis

Another method of informal assessment is task analysis. This technique can be used both for assessment of present level of performance and for instructional planning. Task analysis is defined as identifying the components of a skill or movement and ordering them in a sequence (Dunn and Fait, 1989). Conducting a task analysis involves three steps: (1) breaking down the behavior into essential subtasks, (2) arranging the subtasks in sequence, and (3) describing each subtask in the sequence as an instructional objective.

Task analysis is valuable in planning and breaking down instruction into a sequence of teachable units. As an informal assessment technique, it can be used when skills are problematic for an individual. The skill is analyzed in a sequence of subtasks (or submovements). The ability to perform each submovement is then assessed to discover at which steps of the sequence additional instruction is needed. The *I CAN* program is an example of a physical education program based on task analysis. Task analysis can be used as a type of assessment to identify submovements which then become the objectives for which criterion-referenced tests are developed.

Presently Davis and Burton (1991) advocate an alternative to traditional task analysis by including the components of the task, environment, and performance. Included in Table 5.3 are the functional movement task categories as they relate to movement skills (Davis and Burton, 1991, p. 162). Each part of task

TABLE 5.3 Functional Movement Task Categories and Related Movement Skills

Functional Task Categories	Related Movement Skills
Locomotion: to move from one place to another Criteria: to move with efficiency, precision, accuracy, speed, and/or distance	Roll, crawl/creep, walk/ run, jump/hop/leap, slide/glide, climb, swim
Locomotion on object: to move on a self-propelled object one place to another Criteria: to move with efficiency, precision, accuracy, speed, and/or distance	Propel bicycle, propel boat/canoe, propel skateboard/scooter, propel skates/skis, propel wheelchair
Propulsion: to propel a stationary or moving object or person Criteria: to propel with efficiency, precision, accuracy, speed, and/or distance	Carry, drop, lift, pull-push (bounce, dribble), strike (bat, kick, hit), throw
Reception: to take or receive a (a) stationary or (b) moving object or person Criteria: to secure in hands, feet or other body part or in an implement (e.g., glove, net), bring to a halt at a close proximity to self	(a) Grasp, (b) catch, (b) block
Orientation: (a) to change position of body or body part relative to an object, person, terrain, or event, or (b) to change position of an object or person relative to body or body part or object Criteria: to move with efficiency, speed, accuracy, and/or precision	(a) Bend (lean), (a) reach, (a) turn, (a) twist, (b) manipulate, (b) write/color/draw

From Davis and Burton, 1991. Used with permission.

analysis can be helpful as long as it relates to providing needed information and developing appropriate teaching or family service plans.

Other Informal Assessment Methods

Other types of informal motor tests include checklists, rating scales, interviews, and questionnaires. These assessment procedures incorporate techniques that allow access to otherwise unobservable behaviors such as attitudes, opinions, or medical history.

Checklists

Checklists provide a method of informal assessment in educational or home-based settings. Teachers and/or parents can quickly scan a descriptive list of motor or fitness behaviors and check the appropriate responses that apply. Developmental profiles are often in a checklist format with the basic assumption being that the tester has carefully observed the individual and can accurately describe the current or past behavior. Checklists also provide an excellent format for gathering information not readily available in the educational or clinical setting by collecting valuable information from parents, physicians, or therapists about the individual's developmental history and medical concerns. Further, information from former teachers and other professionals can be gathered by means of checklists to document long range changes in functioning.

Rating Scales

Other informal assessment tools are rating scales. Rating scales enable the tester to express opinions and judgments, as well as evaluate or rate a performance, instead of merely reporting observations. A basic assumption is that the tester has carefully observed the individual and is able to form accurate, professional judgments. One common type of rating scale is a numerical scale based on the premise that 1 means low or poor performance, 3 means average or acceptable performance, and 5 means high or superior performance for the student's/client's age. Rating scales are sometimes useful in assessing attitudes. Progress can also be recorded on a rating scale with: (a) improvement shown, (b) improvement needed, and so forth. This type of rating scale is used frequently on report cards in which no letter grade is given.

Interviews and Questionnaires

Interviews and questionnaires are two methods of informal assessment designed to amass facts and gather information about opinions and attitudes. Interviews are conducted orally while questionnaires primarily call for written responses. There are wide varieties of interviews and questionnaires, from the highly structured to those that are open-ended and flexible enough to allow for further exploration of relevant topics. Interviews and questionnaires can be designed to tap several different physical education domains, such as social interaction and physical performance, and may be designed for individuals with varying levels of ability. Like other informal assessment procedures, interviews and questionnaires have an underlying assumption that the tester has accurately gathered and recorded the information and will report the information correctly. Questionnaires are useful in gathering information from parents about the child's medical history, birth history, infant development, and other developmental history. Interviews and questionnaires can also be used to gather information directly, such as opinions about an individual's performance or activity.

Interpreting Informal Tests

Informal assessment tools, including checklists, rating scales, and questionnaires, do not directly measure behavior, but are instead dependent on information gathered from the informants. The value of that information hinges on the accuracy of information provided by the informant. Problems in using informal measures include incorrect memory of past events, inadequate observation of current events, and faulty judgments.

Interpretation of informal test results should be based on the quality of the informal procedure. Any criterion established for interpreting informal results is selected judgmentally, and that makes translation into meaningful instruction difficult. Furthermore, most informal tests sample only a few skills. Informal assessment can provide a valuable component of the comprehensive assessment.

Informal assessment is a valuable complement to formal, standardized tests. For example, if standardized test results reveal that functional ability is below average range for a particular age level, then informal assessment procedures such as criterion-referenced tests and checklists can provide vital information about the specific skills acquired and those tasks or goals for which special instruction is needed. In this manner, informal tests can assist in a comprehensive assessment process by providing information that cannot be generated by a formal testing procedure.

Norm-Referenced Tests

As discussed in Chapter Two, tests that examine an individual's performance in relation to the performance of a representative group are norm-referenced tests. Norm-referenced tests are frequently confused with "formal tests" and "standardized tests." Norm-referenced tests are a kind of formal test while a standardized test is one in which all children are given the same tasks under uniform directions. In norm-referenced tests, "norm" refers to the test performance of a sample of subjects with characteristics similar to those subjects for whom the test was designed (for example, 8-year-old girls of mixed races from a range of economic backgrounds and from all geographic areas).

A norm-referenced motor test is used when a teacher wants to administer a test that determines with great accuracy the children who have high, average, and low motor proficiency. If a teacher wants to determine the relative position (high or low) of a child's motor skill performance in relation to others with similar characteristics, the teacher should select a well-constructed norm-referenced test as the appropriate instrument. Norm-referenced tests can be useful tools for guiding placement decisions in the least restrictive environment.

A norm-referenced motor test is designed to determine an individual's rank-order position in relation to the motor performance of a norm group (peers) who have also taken the test. To be an accurate assessment of an individual's relative position, a wide range of motor performances must be included. A norm-referenced motor test is constructed around the author's choice of components for the motor domain. The Physical Best Fitness Test, for example, contains items designed to test physical fitness, while the Bruininks-Oseretsky Test was developed to assess overall motor proficiency. Norm-referenced tests are usually developed to assess general areas of motor and/or fitness performance, rather than specific skill.

The challenge for the development of a test is to develop clear, reliable, and valid test items representing the particular attitudes of motor performance to be assessed. Once test items are developed, they must then be piloted on a sample of subjects representative of those for whom the test is being designed. When the data from the sample has been collected, it is analyzed item by item to determine which items to retain. The best items are judged to be those that produce the greatest diversity of scores. Items that were responded to either correctly or incorrectly by too many subjects are usually eliminated. Baumgartner and Jackson (1995) noted that the test items should be unrelated and not affect other items in a test battery, be able to discriminate among ability groups and be specific to what is being measured. Also, tests should reflect performances of individuals as they receive instruction in that area. For example, if the Baumgartner Pull-Up Test is used to measure strength, instruction should not include training on the pull-up but on other aspects of instruction to induce strength gains that can be measured by this test.

Following this procedure, the revised test is administered to a group of students representative of those for whom the test was designed (norm group). Lastly, studies of reliability and validity are conducted on the final version of the test.

Statistics of Norm-Referenced Tests

A norm-referenced test is based on the assumption that behaviors are normally distributed. Three measures of central tendency describe the sample distribution of test scores: the mean, mode, and median. These three terms refer to typical, or average, performance. Teachers who wish to examine how well a group of children generally performed will use the mode, which is the most frequently occurring score. To determine the midpoint of a distribution, a teacher calculates the median, the point at which half of the scores are higher and half are lower. The median is helpful in describing distributions that contain a few unusually high or low scores. Most often the mean is used to describe the central tendency of a distribution. The mean is actually the arithmetic average of a distribution, obtained by summing the scores and dividing the sum by the number of scores. When using measures of central tendency, remember that these terms are appropriate for describing a group but are not necessarily useful in describing an individual group member since a few extreme scores can distract the distribution.

Measures of validity describe how much the scores in a distribution vary from one another. The most common description of variability in an educational setting is the standard deviation, a calculation based on the degree to which the scores deviate from the mean. We refer to a score as being a certain number of standard deviations above (+) or greater than the mean, or a certain number below (–) or less than the mean. In normal distributions, a precise relationship exists between the standard deviation and the percentage of students whose scores fall within 1 standard deviation above or below the mean. For any normal distribution, 68.2 percent of the scores will be between +1 standard deviation and –1 standard deviation.

Standard deviations can be useful in determining cutoff points for placement in the least restrictive environment. A school district may decide, for example, that a score of 2 deviations below the mean on a norm-referenced skills test along with other vital assessment information meets the criteria for eligibility. However, placement does not always satisfy program planning and the needs of the child. Specific criteria must be established to present an adequate picture of the student's/client's functional ability.

Norm-Referenced Test Scores

The number of correct responses on a test constitutes the raw scores that are basic to calculating descriptive data. In norm-referenced tests, raw scores take on meaning when they are compared with the scores of individuals in the norm group. The result of this comparison is a type of source called a norm, which is a description of the performance of that specific group. When discussing norm-referenced test scores, the normal curve is used to illustrate the relationship of the types of scores to one another and to the curve.

Percentile Norms

Percentile norms are used frequently when reporting educational diagnostic data. A percentile norm tells the percentage of a norm group that falls at or below a specific score. If an individual received a raw score of 20, which the test norms indicate is better than 45 percent of the norm group, then the percentile rank is 45.

One of the advantages of using percentiles is that they are relatively easy to understand. Individuals unfamiliar with testing procedures can readily understand that a percentile of 45 means that a child demonstrated near-average performance as compared with the norm group. Another advantage of using percentile norms is that the norm-reference group has characteristics similar to those of the student taking the test. On the Physical Best Fitness Test, for example, the score of a 12-year-old girl is based on a comparison with the 12-year-old girls in the norm group. For each age group for which the test is designed, a set of percentile norms should be available. A third advantage of percentile scores is that they can be easily used to compare a child's performance in several subtest areas or across various subject areas. Percentile scores on a motor ability test, for example, can be examined with percentile scores in reading and mathematics achievement. A child who is at the 10th percentile in motor ability, the 60th percentile in reading, and the 45th in mathematics, demonstrates relatively low motor performance compared with other subject areas.

One caution should be noted, however, when using percentile scores: a percentile norm does not have equal units at all points on the scale. For example, percentiles of 45 on speed and agility and 53 on balance represent very similar raw scores. In contrast, the same 5-point difference at the 2nd and 7th percentiles represents correspondingly large differences. A distribution that closely approximates normality should reveal a clustering of percentile scores toward the middle of the distribution. However, it should be remembered that percentiles cannot be averaged on various components.

Standard Scores

Standard score norms describe the distance of a child's test score from the mean in terms of standard deviations. Examples of standard scores are T scores and Z scores. Another standard score that is used more frequently in educational settings is the stanine score. Stanine scores have a mean of 5 and a standard deviation of approximately 2. Like percentile scores, standard scores carry uniform size characteristics from test to test. Standard scores should be used with caution, however, because in some tests the scores are contaminated by other variables, such as grade-basing rather than age-basing.

Developmental Norms

Developmental norms, or age-score norms, are particularly meaningful because they indicate how far along the normal motor developmental continuum an individual has progressed. Developmental norms can provide information such as whether a 6-year-old boy's current motor behavior is approximately like that of other 6-year-old boys. Developmental information is being increasingly emphasized in assessment in developmental programs. Determining a given child's fitness or motor skill development level provides vital information in fashioning individualized programs. Because developmental scores do not carry uniform meaning from test to test and are not of uniform size, their usefulness is somewhat limited for purposes of comparisons.

Criterion-Referenced Tests

Criterion-referenced tests have become increasingly popular in recent educational and behavioral psychology settings. While norm-referenced tests indicate an individual's relative status in motor and fitness development in comparison with a peer sample, criterion-referenced motor tests measure motor skill development in terms of absolute levels of mastery. Criterion-referenced tests compare performance to some predetermined criterion, rather than to the performance of others. These tests are usually curriculum-based, to determine which skills have been mastered. Criterion-referenced tests simply measure the aspects of motor and fitness behavior that an individual can and cannot accomplish. The tests do not provide information about what is average performance based on the age of the individual.

Criterion-referenced tests are relatively easy to construct, can be used to measure any behavior, and are directly relevant to instruction. Specific instructional questions are used to generate criterion-referenced tests. For example, a recreation leader may want to know if John can dribble a ball ten times consecutively, demonstrate accuracy in a volleyball service, or complete 25 repetitions of an exercise. Any of these questions can be answered by constructing a criterion-referenced test. King and Aufsesser (1988) suggested the following guidelines for developing criterion-referenced tests:

1. Decide what specific questions you want answered about an individual's performance.
2. Write a performance objective that describes how you are going to test the child, including conditions, specific behavior, and criteria for acceptance.
3. Use performance objectives to develop the criterion-referenced test, including directions, scoring, and equipment.

Questions about the individual's functional capabilities form the basis for developing a criterion-referenced test. These questions may be generated from: (1) performance in general motor or fitness areas on a norm-referenced test, (2) analysis and observation of a child's performance during class, play, or clinical settings, or (3) class records of progress.

Once the questions are formulated in specific terms, they are used to write performance objectives. Performance objectives should include:

1. Desired behavior stated in observable terms
2. Conditions under which the behavior should occur
3. Criterion for acceptable performance

For example, a physical education teacher may be interested in determining if a child can "kick a ball." This is an important question, but it needs to be further defined. "Kicking a ball" can be interpreted as a toe-kick, a kick for distance, a kick for accuracy, or a soccer dribble. The question should be specifically stated to describe the skill the teacher is interested in, such as: The child, when requested by the teacher to "kick the ball," will kick a 10-inch ball into a 6-foot-wide, 3-foot-high goal area, using a shoelace kick, from a distance of 12 feet, four out of five times.

The criterion in this objective is "four out of five times." The criterion can be determined by identifying same-aged individuals who possess the skill desired and measuring their performance against the objective. The minimum level of performance by these children then becomes the standard for passing that item on a criterion-referenced test.

The *I CAN* program (Kelly and Wessel, 1976) uses performance objectives. Each objective is tested by means of a criterion-referenced assessment. If a child passes a criterion-referenced item, the teacher can assume that the child has mastered the performance objective assessed by the test, and instruction may then progress to the next objective in the curriculum sequence. When a child does not pass a criterion-referenced item, testing should continue until the child passes an objective (usually lower in sequence) to determine the next objective for instruction.

Teachers may design their own criterion-referenced tests to fit their instructional program, or they may use a commercially prepared curriculum such as the *I CAN* program that includes assessment items. The Data-Based Gymnasium (Dunn, 1986) also contains criterion-referenced motor tests that are useful in writing individualized education programs. Likewise, Bricker (1993) recently published

AEPS: Measurement for Birth to Three Years, a criterion-referenced instrument to evaluate preschool children's progress on selected goals and to make comparisons to previous performances.

Statistics from Criterion-Referenced Tests

The quality of criterion-referenced tests is generally unknown and difficult to measure. Because of their highly skill-specific nature and predominantly local usage, few data are available on standardization, reliability, or validity. The *I CAN* program has been nationally validated and studies of reliability have been conducted. A further attempt to standardize criterion-referenced physical education test items has been undertaken by Ulrich (1986) in the *Test of Gross Motor Development* (TGMD).

Criterion-Referenced Test Scores

Scores derived from criterion-referenced tests are directly interpretable to the specified terms. Because criterion-referenced tests contain "standards," the scale common to these tests is the percentage of items correct. The administration and scoring of criterion-referenced tests should also be explicit and objective to ensure that all individuals are judged according to the same standard (King and Aufsesser, 1988). Test scores generally specify the percentage of items in a domain that have been performed and are essentially raw. The raw scores obtained from criterion-referenced tests are meaningful if the motor content and the test specification are described as clearly and precisely as possible. In criterion-referenced tests, no derived scores are calculated because normative comparisons are not made. Although the reliability of criterion-referenced tests may not be specified, it is important to determine the reliability of these measures by utilizing several data points or objectivity ratings discussed earlier.

Judging Technical Adequacy

Since many individuals with disabilities form a heterogeneous group, the limited availability of a variety of tests may be frustrating. Not only are teachers and recreation leaders required to individualize instruction, but test selection requires teachers/leaders to be skilled in judging the technical adequacy of tests. It is essential to seek reviews of specific instruments for evaluating tests, such as *Tests in Print IV* and the *Mental Measurements Yearbook* (Buros Institute, 1992; supplement 1994) and *Assessment in Special and Remedial Education* (Salvia and Ysseldyke, 1991), as well as reviews in clinical and educational journals. All provide valuable guidelines for judging the technical merit of assessment instruments. Some resources may focus primarily on psychological and academic tests and provide only scant reviews of tests in the psychomotor domain. Although such resources have limitations, the challenge is to be as critical and precise as possible when administering tests, understanding and interpreting results, and making decisions based on test results. Not all tests will be appropriate for every situation and should be selected on their appropriateness and ability to generate useful information for program planning or evaluation. Test users should review their skills according to the following qualifications:

1. Have a general knowledge of measurement principles and the limitations of test interpretations
2. Be qualified to administer and interpret specific tests
3. Decision making should come from an understanding of measurement procedures and its validation
4. Specific training is needed to administer and interpret test scores. Anyone administering a test of motor skill development for decision-making purposes should be competent to administer the test. If unqualified, necessary training should be sought regardless of previous educational training
5. Test users should seek to avoid biased or discriminatory practices in test selection, administration, and interpretation (especially bias of age, sex, cultural background, or condition)
6. Consistent administration practices should be employed by the tester

When it appears that a test does not meet the standards of technical adequacy, several courses of action can be taken. If the test is inadequate in validity, reliability, and standardization, it cannot be used. The test may, however, contain specific items that are useful if administered individually. If, for example, you believe that a particular item testing balance would be helpful, the item can be administered if precautions are followed. First, check the validity to see if the item does indeed test what you want it to test (e.g., dynamic balance). Second, determine the interrater reliability for the item by calculating percentage of agreement. The item can be administered and scored by other testers or on different occasions to check reliability. Third, the intrarater reliability should also be determined to ascertain stability reliability on several days. Baumgartner and Jackson (1995) indicated that low stability reliability can occur when (1) people tested perform differently, (2) the measuring instrument operates differently, and (3) the person administering the test varies. Fourth, do not report the results of a single item comparatively if the standardization sample is inadequate. These guidelines can also be used for tests that are inadequate in one of the areas of validity, reliability, or standardization. If a test is reliable and valid but has an inadequate standardization sample for a given child, then comparison results should not be computed. The test user should examine instead the differences between the characteristics of the student to be tested and the characteristics of the individuals on whom the test norms were developed. The tester's responsibility is to decide whether the differences are so great that the test should not be used for that student.

The guidelines suggested should be followed when selecting, administering, or interpreting tests and when transmitting such interpretations to others. It is vital to remember that scores on tests must never be interpreted as representing innate, fixed abilities and characteristics of the individual being tested. Also important is the recognition that measurement error exists in any test score and must be taken into account in test interpretations. Lastly, be sure to provide test interpretations that are

TABLE 5.4 Checklist Results Used to Determine an Assessment Battery

Checklist Information	Types of Assessment
1. *Purpose of assessment?* Instructional planning	Criterion-referenced tests, informal tests.
2. *Components of program?* Fundamental motor skills Physical fitness Participation	Rating scales based on observation or video-tape. Baseline endurance rate, and evaluation of range of motion and functional capabilities. Observation of social integration, amount of movement, general attitude toward activity.
3. *Characteristics?* Average intellectually Shy, self-concious	Assessment should provide success and reinforcement.
Cerebral palsy, lower extremity, hip, knee, ankle spasticity. Wears short leg braces and uses quadruped canes.	Use normal task analyses for upper extremities, except where balance may interfere. Parent interview. Reports of physician, physical therapist. Interview classroom teacher. Observe classes, playground, recreational setting. Most important is determination of level of play, participation and amount of physical activity in natural environments.

based on technically adequate scores, are clear, and are readily understandable by other members of the child-study team.

When No Appropriate Tests Are Available

Because of the wide variation among individuals with disabilities, no single test or criterion can be adequate for everyone. Not surprisingly, the test user will not always find a single test that seems appropriate. Likewise, tests are not always useful in determining specific needs of the individual. The evaluator still has the responsibility, however, of gathering the appropriate information and assessments that provide meaningful information for decision making and program planning.

Table 5.4 presents a systematic checklist for developing an appropriate assessment battery. The first step in conducting this assessment is to establish clearly defined motor or fitness objectives that fulfill the purpose of the assessment. Next, the characteristics of the individual are taken into consideration. Relevant cognitive, affective, and physical characteristics that affect the assessment should be considered. The results of the checklist can lead to the selection of an individualized assessment battery as demonstrated in Table 5.4 by completing the checklist for a child with cerebral palsy.

The complex, individualized nature of assessment of individuals with disabilities is evident in this example. Assessment is a multifaceted process that may or may not include commercially available tests, and when formal tests are not available, informal measures become the vital instruments for information gathering.

References

Baumgartner, T., and A. Jackson. *Measurement for Evaluation in Physical Education,* 5th ed. Dubuque, IA: Brown and Benchmark, 1995.

Bricker, D. *AEPS: Measurement for Birth to Three Years* (Vol. 1) Baltimore, MD: P. H. Brookes Publishing Co., 1993.

Buros Institute. *Mental Measurements Yearbook.* Lincoln: University of Nebraska, 1992.

Buros Institute. *Tests in Print IV.* Lincoln: University of Nebraska, 1994.

Davis, W. E., and A. W. Burton. "Ecological Task Analysis: Translating Movement Behavior Theory into Practice." *Adapted Physical Activity Quarterly, 8*(2), 1991, 154–177.

Dunn, J. M. *The Data-Based Gymnasium: A Systematic Approach to Physical Education for the Handicapped.* Austin, TX: Pro-Ed, 1986.

Dunn and Fait. *Special Physical Education: Adapted Individualized Developmental,* 6th ed. 1989.

Fernhall, B., and G. Tymeson. "Graded Exercise Testing of Mentally Retarded Adults: A Study of Feasibility." *Archives of Physical Medicine and Rehabilitation* 68, 1987, 363–365.

Horvat, M., R. Croce, and G. Roswal. "Magnitude and Reliability of Measurements of Muscle Strength Across Trials for Individuals with Mental Retardation." *Perceptual and Motor Skills, 77,* 1993, 643–649.

Horvat, M., B. G. McManis, and F. E. Seagraves. "Reliability and Objectivity of the Nicholas Manual Muscle Tester with Children." *Isokinetics and Exercise Science, 21*(4), 1992, 175–181.

Kelly, L., and J. A. Wessel. *I CAN: Primary Skills.* Austin, TX: Pro-Ed, 1990.

King, L., and K. Aufsesser. "Criterion-Referenced Testing: An Ongoing Process." *Journal of Physical Education, Recreation and Dance, 59,* 1988, 58–63.

Salvia, J., and J. E. Ysseldyke. *Assessment in Special and Remedial Education,* 5th ed. Boston: Houghton Mifflin Co., 1991.

Schmidt, L. S., S. L. Westcott, and T. K. Crowe. "Interrater Reliability of the Gross Motor Scale of the Peabody Developmental Motor Scales with Four- and Five-Year-Old Children." *Pediatric Physical Therapy, 5*(4), 1993, 169–175.

Ulrich, D. *Test of Gross Motor Development.* Austin, TX: Pro-Ed, 1986.

CHAPTER 6

Motor Skill and Development

The focus of overall development should provide relevant information related to placement and the determination of functional capabilities of individuals with disabilities. Several sources of information contribute to identifying specific developmental landmarks, reflex movements, and voluntary movements that are used for ambulation, stability, and object control. Later these movements become patterns and are used in conjunction with other movements to accomplish specific tasks or are performed in recreational activities on an individual basis or competitive format. In this chapter, the focus will be on development of movement and coordination, including tests of motor development, reflexes, motor ability, perceptual motor, coordination, and sport skill assessments.

Motor development tests are designed to evaluate progression of normal motor functioning on a continuum. The use of developmental norms assumes that comparing the performance of an individual with disabilities to normal development is appropriate and deviations from the norm are indicative of a delay, a problem in development, or are associated with a physical or learning disability. Developmental scores, including age and grade equivalents, compare performances across age or grade peer groups and are useful in clinical case studies, initial motor development screening, detecting potential movement dysfunctions, and in longitudinal research on motor development. The use of a developmental approach assumes that all individuals progress through the same series of motor developmental tasks, although they may encounter landmarks at various time intervals in the developmental process.

Reflex Tests

Reflexes are involuntary subcortical movements that are exhibited by responses to the environment and provide measurement protection and information gathering functions (Horvat, 1990). Although primarily associated with infants and their earliest movements because of the undeveloped neurological system, it is apparent that neurological dysfunctions at any age may disrupt motor functioning or provide false positives concerning the strength of a muscle group. For example, initiation of the *asymmetrical* or *symmetrical tonic neck reflex* may cause alternate flexion or extension of the extremities that can disrupt the stability of the individual. Likewise, a *startle reflex* may cause the infant to fall while in a quadrupedal position.

In most school, recreational, clinical, or sport settings, reflex assessments are not commonly performed unless the individual has persistent neurological problems. However, the awareness of persistent reflex behavior is imperative to understanding if the reflex is contributing to or detracting from the performance. For example, inappropriate movements that will initiate a reflex can be avoided, such as neck flexion, while proper strategies, such as strengthening neck muscles, can be implemented to avoid some reflex actions. For individuals with disabilities, one should identify the level of functioning and then provide appropriate tasks to facilitate reflex inhibition.

Sherrill (1993) contends that of all the reflexes that affect motor behavior, only ten principal reflexes are closely aligned to movement performance. These include: (a) hand grasp reflex, (b) asymmetrical tonic neck reflex, (c) moro reflex, (d) symmetrical tonic neck reflex, (e) foot grasp reflex, (f) tonic labyrinthine reflex—supine, (g) tonic labyrinthine reflex—prone, (h) crossed extension reflex, (i) extensor thrust reflex, and (j) positive support reflex. Spinal level reflexes are concerned with protection and nourishment of the infant, such as the crossed extension and extensor thrust. Brain stem reflexes, such as tonic neck, labyrinthine, and associated reactions, are tuning reflexes that affect muscle tone rather than produce specific movements. In addition, other reactions or reflexes could appear during infancy and early childhood. These remain throughout the life span, and provide righting or protective reactions that allow the infant to assume some movement control and coordinate various body positions, such as lifting the head and turning the body. These righting reactions are higher levels of functions of neurological development that maintain the head in the upright posture and align the head, neck, and trunk. If the head and neck do not follow the body, movement is impeded. Further, as the body is tilted, protective reactions are elicited to compensate for changes in position and to facilitate muscle tone. If these adjustments are not made, standing ambulation and reciprocal leg movements are affected. Commonly, this is demonstrated by a lack of balance or inability to perform basic motor skills. Equilibrium reactions are used to maintain balance in response to changes in the center of gravity or base of support (O'Sullivan and Schmitz, 1988). These are evaluated by equilibrium platforms or gymnastic balls to assess tilting reactions and the individual's adjustments to maintain balance.

Scoring of reflexes is generally subjective with a scoring key to denote absence or changes in the movement. Scoring may range from 0 or normal to 1—decreased, 2—absent, 3—exaggerated, or 4—sustained. Several common developmental reflexes that may be helpful in determining potential motor behavior problems are included in Table 6.1 (Haywood, 1993; O'Sullivan and Schmitz, 1988).

TABLE 6.1 Common Reflexes Used to Identify Motor Problems

Reflex (Reaction)	Stimulus	Response	Persistence
Brain stem reflexes Asymmetrical tonic neck reflex	Rotation or lateral flexion of the head.	Increased extension on chin side with accompanying flexion of limbs on head side.	Difficulty in rolling because of extended arm; interferes with holding the head in midline resulting in problems with tracking and fixating on objects. Evident in catching and throwing when one elbow is bent while the other extends because head position rotates or tilts to track a ball.
Symmetrical tonic neck reflex	Flexion or extension of the head and neck.	With head flexion flexes arms and upper extremities with extension of the legs. Backward extension of head results in extension of arms and flexion of legs.	Prevents creeping because head controls position of arms and legs. Retention prohibits infants from flexing and extending legs in creeping patterns. Also interferes with catching, kicking, and throwing since changes in head position affect muscle tone and reciprocation of muscle groups.
Tonic labyrinthine (prone and supine)	Stimulation of vestibular apparatus by tilting or changes in head position.	In prone position increased flexion in the limbs, while in supine position extension occurs in limbs.	Affects muscle tone and ability to move body segments independently into various positions such as propping the body up in a support position prior to crawling or rolling.

TABLE 6.1—*Continued*

Reflex (Reaction)	Stimulus	Response	Persistence
Positive support	Stimulation when the balls of the feet touch a firm surface in an upright position.	Extension of the legs to support individual's weight in a standing position.	Disruption of muscle tone needed to support weight or adduction and internal rotation of the hips that interferes with standing and locomotion.
Spinal reflexes Grasping reflex (Palmar and Plantar grasping)	Pressure on palm of hand or hypertension of wrist. Plantar grasping, stroking the sole of foot will initiate contraction of toes.	Flexion of fingers to grasp then extension to release. In foot, toes contract around object stroking foot.	In hand causes difficulty in releasing objects, in throwing and in striking, and in reception of tactile stimuli. In foot interferes with static and dynamic balance while standing and walking.
Crossed extension reflex	Stimulation to ball of foot.	Flexion followed by extension and adduction of opposite leg.	Coordination of leg movements in creeping and walking impeded by stiffness and lack of reciprocal leg movement.
Extensor thrust reflex	Sudden pressure or prick to sole of foot in sitting or supine position.	Toes extend foot dorsiflexes with increased extensor tone.	Balance between flexion and extension impeded, often seen as stiffness of body in sitting position.
Moro reflex	Change in head position; drop backward in a sitting position.	Arms and legs extend, fingers spread; then arms flex, addition of arms across chest.	Interferes with ability to sit unsupported and locomotor patterns or sports skills with sudden movements, i.e., abduction of arms and legs during gymnastics interferes with balance.

TABLE 6.1—*Continued*

Postural Reactions	Stimulus	Response	Persistence
Body righting	Rotate upper or lower trunk.	Body segment that is not rotated allows to align body.	Interferes with ability to right itself when head is held in a lateral position.
Neck righting	Turn head sideways.	Body follows head in rotation.	Cannot align head with neck when body is turned. Impedes segmental rolling.
Labyrinthine righting	Limit vision or tilt body in various directions.	Head will move to maintain upright position.	Unable to reorient head in proper body alignment and position. Interferes with head control in movement.
Optic righting	Tilt body in various directions.	Allows head to achieve upright position.	Unable to reorient head in proper body alignment and body posture. Interferes with head control in movement.
Parachute reactions	Lower infant forward rapidly or tilt forward to prone position.	Legs and arms extend and abduct to protect from fall.	Lack of support to prevent body from falling.
Tilting reactions	Displace center of gravity by tilting or moving support surface.	Protective extension and muscle tone on downward side. Upward side has curvature of trunk and extension and abduction of extremities.	Clumsiness and awkwardness resulting in loss of balance, muscle tone and falling.

Adapted from O'Sullivan and Schmitz, *Physical Rehabilitation: Assessment and Treatment*, 2nd ed. Reproduced with permission of F.A. Davis Company.

Other Reflex Tests

Milani-Comparetti Neuromotor Developmental Examination

The Milani-Comparetti assessment is available in most settings to evaluate the neurological maturity of infants from birth to 24 months in two areas: spontaneous behavior and evolved responses (Milani-Comparetti and Gidoni, 1967). Spontaneous behaviors include many developmental landmarks such as head control, body control, and active movements such as standing. Infants from birth to 24 months are assessed for primitive reflexes, righting, parachute, and tilting reactions. Scoring ranges from 1 to 5 points with 5 indicative of typical functioning, 3 to 4 indicative of mild to moderate abnormal functioning, and 1 to 2 indicative of severe dysfunction. Assessment is related to months that reflexes or reactions should occur given typical development. Sherrill (1993) recommends that outside a clinical setting, absence or presence of a landmark reflex or reaction should be noted using the letters "A" or "P" as appropriate. Payne and Issacs (1995) feel this assessment is suitable to monitor motor functioning during medical checkups and is useful in children with motor delays.

Florentino Reflex Test

Florentino has long been associated with reflex testing in typical and atypical development (Florentino, 1972). The focus of the Florentino Reflex Test is directly related to understanding and analysis of factors that contribute to atypical development through the retention of primitive reflexes. This test is especially useful for individuals with severe involvement and for individuals with cerebral palsy. A criterion-referenced plus (+) or minus (–) score indicates presence or absence of a reflex or reaction that may result in abnormal muscle tone and positive or negative motor delays.

Primitive Reflex Profile

An instrument developed by Capute et al. (1984) quantifiably assesses primitive reflex behaviors (asymmetrical tonic neck, symmetrical tonic neck, and the Moro reflex). The scale, which follows, employs a 5-point classification scoring system to observe typical and atypical movement responses and note the strength of the reflex. Primitive reflexes were selected, being the most indicative of atypical development.

0 = absent
1 = small change in tone
2 = physically present and visible
3 = noticeable strength and force
4 = strong

Motor Development Tests

A major premise in motor development is that certain behaviors emerge through maturational processes and then develop through learning and practice. Problems may interfere with this process, the result being that children may fail to achieve appropriate developmental landmarks. For the educator or parent, these normally expected milestones are cues to potential problems in development. For the teacher or recreational leader, they facilitate identification of entry levels for intervention and program planning. Some of the common tests used to assess developmental landmarks follow.

Denver II

The Denver II (see Figure 6.1) is a revision of the Denver Developmental Screening Test (Frankenburg, Goldstein, and Camp, 1975) to assess development in children ages 0–6 years (Frankenburg, Dodds, and Archer, 1990). By design, the test is simple, quick to administer, and inexpensive. It assesses development in four areas:

1. Gross motor (e.g., sitting, walking, broad jumping, throwing a ball overhand, balancing on one foot)
2. Fine motor-adaptive (e.g., stacking blocks, reaching for objects, drawing a person)
3. Language (e.g., responding to sounds, imitating speech sounds, recognizing colors, counting)
4. Personal-social (e.g., smiling responsively, feeding self, dressing)

The Denver II contains 125 items, with approximately 32 items on the gross motor scale, and proceeds in a developmental progression. Each child is tested individually and is scored as pass, fail, refusal, or no opportunity (due to parent or guardian restrictions). The norms show a range of ages by month during which a particular behavior could appear. The norms include charts that reflect the age at which 25, 50, 75, and 90 percent of the children can achieve certain behaviors. The child would be "delayed" on those items for which achievement does not compare with age group peers. Children who demonstrate one or more delays on the test are considered for further evaluation.

The original version of the test was criticized for being unrepresentative because of its standardization sample and test reliability (Werder and Kalakian, 1985). The revision of the test includes stability reliability and interrater reliability that is between 80–100 percent for most items. Validity of the Denver II was based on a regression analysis and standardization data of more than 2,000 subjects (Frankenburg, Dodds, Archer, Shapiro, and Bresnick, 1992). This version has overcome many of the original concerns of the DDST and is a valuable screening tool for young children with developmental delays.

Bayley Scales of Infant Development (Bayley II)

The revision of *Bayley Scales of Infant Development* (2nd ed., 1993) is the revision of the 1969 Bayley Scales designed to determine current developmental status and the extent of deviations from expected peer group development. The Bayley II provides a three-part evaluation of the developmental states of infants and preschoolers at risk: Mental Scale (sensory-perceptual acuities, discrimination), Motor Scale (fine and gross), and Behavior Rating Scale (attention/arousal, orientation/engagement, emotional regulation, motor quality). The Motor Scale results are expressed

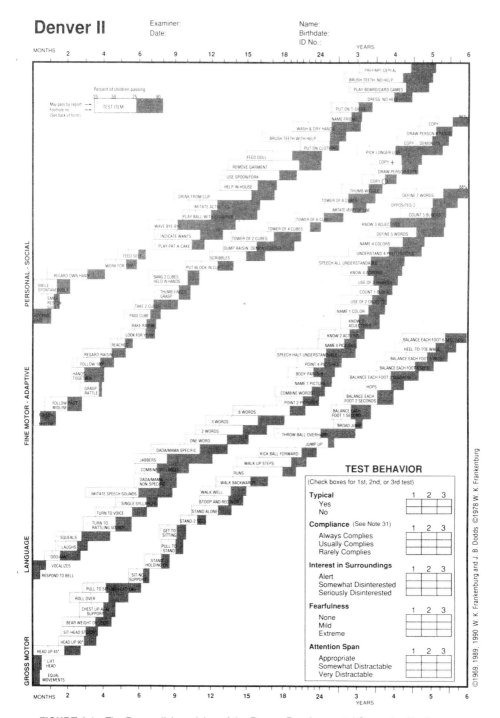

FIGURE 6.1 The Denver II (a revision of the Denver Developmental Screening Test)

From Frankenburg, W.K. Used with permission of Denver Developmental Materials. P.O. Box 6919, Denver, CO, 80205–8919.

as a standard score (Psychomotor Development Index) measuring body control, large muscle coordination, finger manipulation, dynamic movement, dynamic praxis, postural imitation, and stereognosis.

The Bayley II was renormed on a sample of 1700 (850 boys, 850 girls), ages 1 month to 42 months in 1-month intervals. As a departure from the earlier stated design of assessing normal motor development, the primary use of the current Bayley Scales is with at-risk children or those who are expected to be at risk (Bayley, 1993). It is reported in the Instructional Manual that information regarding validity was extrapolated from clinical samples and with at-risk children who are premature, have the HIV antibody, are prenatally drug exposed, asphyxiated at birth, developmentally delayed, have frequent otitis media, are autistic, or have Down's syndrome (Bayley, 1993).

The test manual is clearly written and provides normative data to compare performance with age group peers as well as provide the clinician with follow-up evaluations. Test administration is suggested for a single session or two sessions if needed. The scoring procedures allow the examiner to determine a child's developmental age for each domain (Bayley, 1993). Score possibilities include pass, fail, or other (omitted, refused, or reported by parent) with subsequent conversions to the Developmental Index. In contrast to the Denver II, the Bayley II is a more expensive test requiring construction of some special equipment and stimulus materials. However, Bayley II appears to be a welcome revision of the developmental status of infants, especially children who are at risk for developmental delays. A companion to the Bayley II, the Bayley Infant Neurodevelopmental Screen (BINS) is a screening test designed to measure basic neurological functions, as well as social and cognitive processes, on a pass/fail basis.

Gesell Developmental Schedules (GDS)

Gesell Developmental Schedules (Gesell and Amatruda, 1949) compare a list of the child's behaviors with schedules of developmental maturity. They are frequently used to assess the development of infants with early childhood (4 weeks–6 years). The Gesell Developmental Schedules provide developmental information in four areas: motor, adaptive, language, and personal-social. The child's behaviors are compared with the age-level constellations of behaviors in the schedules given on an individual basis. One disadvantage of the instrument is that it is expensive, due in part to the dispersion of vital test information in three different volumes.

Since the Gesell Developmental Schedules were standardized 30 years ago, much of the information may not apply to today's children, especially in light of revisions to the Bayley II and Denver II. In addition, little information is available on test reliability and is not useful because of outdated standardization data, lack of reliability data, and low predictive validity. Therefore, other developmental measures may be more appropriate.

McCarthy Scales of Children's Abilities (MSCA)

The MSCA (McCarthy, 1972) is a norm-referenced test for children 2½–8½ years of age consisting of 18 subtests in the following content areas: Verbal Scale (verbal expression), Perceptual (reasoning ability through manipulation), Quantitative (numbers and vocabulary—Performance Scale), Memory Scale (short-term), Motor Scale (gross and fine), and General Cognitive Scale (overall cognitive functioning). The MSCA is commonly used as an intelligence measure and was standardized on 1,000 nondisabled children.

Pass-fail scoring results in a profile index. The child is classified on a scale to determine general intellectual level as well as weaknesses in areas such as verbal ability and memory (McCarthy, 1972). An adapted version of the MSCA, the McCarthy Screening Test or MST (McCarthy, 1978), can be used to identify children requiring special education assistance in six tests from the original test in the sensorimotor and cognitive domain. These include: Right-Left Acceleration, Verbal Memory (Part 1), Draw a Design, Numerical Memory, and Conceptual Group and Leg Coordination. Although this test is primarily a cognitive measure, the MST can assess abilities of sensorimotor functioning, as well as cognition that may be helpful in identifying learning problems and preferred styles of learning in children.

Early Learning Accomplishment Profiles (E-LAP, LAP, LAP-D)

The Early Learning Accomplishment Profiles (Sanford, 1975) are a series of assessment and programming assessments for children 0–6 years. The E-LAP (0–3 years) assesses gross and fine motor skills, cognition, language, self-help, and social-emotional skills. A profile is developed based on items passed or failed at an approximate age level. The LAP is designed for ages 3–6 and has the same scoring and programming as the E-LAP.

The LAP-D was developed to assess mastery in five areas, including fine motor (manipulation and writing), cognition (matching and counting), language (naming and comprehension), gross motor (body movement and object control), and self-help (eating, grooming, toileting, self-direction). Plus or minus scoring is used to differentiate items completed. All content is alleged to be based on recommendations from experts who have identified landmarks generally associated with development.

Brigance Diagnostic Inventory of Early Development

The Brigance was designed for children from birth to 7 years (Brigance, 1978). The Brigance addresses development in the following areas:

1. Pre-ambulatory motor skills and behaviors
2. Gross motor skills and behaviors
3. Fine motor skills and behaviors
4. Self-help skills
5. Pre-speech
6. Speech and language
7. General knowledge and comprehension
8. Readiness
9. Manuscript writing
10. Mathematics

Scores are recorded as pass-fail for specific items. As long as the child is successful, he or she proceeds until the highest item is completed correctly. The Brigance is also easy to administer and can be implemented in home and school settings. Since the test is widely used by classroom teachers, it can provide useful information on the child's stability and gross motor movement on a criterion basis.

Other Developmental Assessments

Although they do not offer specific formal assessment instruments, two publications contain descriptions of developmental motor patterns for children. Each is an excellent reference and can be used to develop checklists for assessing specific motor patterns that, in turn, can be used to develop program plans. These publications are McClenaghan and Gallahue (1978), *Fundamental Movement,* and Wickstrom (1983), *Fundamental Motor Patterns* (3rd ed.).

The Fundamental Movement Pattern Assessment

The Fundamental Movement Pattern Instrument (McClenaghan and Gallahue, 1978) is an observational assessment used to classify individuals at the initial, elementary, or mature stage of development for throwing, catching, kicking, running, and jumping. Interrater reliability ranges from 80 to 95 percent depending on the pattern assessed and it is a valuable book to assess the quality of a child's movement based on developmental sequences required for fundamental movement abilities (Gallahue, 1989).

Likewise, Wickstrom (1983) evaluates the quality of fundamental movements of walking, running, jumping, throwing, catching, striking, and kicking from beginning to mature patterns. Wickstrom also discusses in-depth information concerning the biomechanics of the developmental patterns and generalization to performance.

Each of these sources is potentially valuable to analyze a specific motor problem of an individual and to develop specific fitness or motor development remediations to facilitate individual development. In addition, each is useful as a checklist of performance indications that are inherent in specific movement patterns.

Motor Ability Tests

Tests of motor ability are designed to provide comparative information about an individual's motor capabilities or proficiencies. Just as intelligence tests assume that a general index of the construct "intelligence" exists, motor ability tests assume the existence of a general index for the construct "motor ability." Furthermore, motor ability tests are designed to be predictive of motor skill performance. They are usually formal tests standardized on representative samples of typically developing subjects at various age levels. Motor ability tests are administered for the following reasons:

1. To determine general motor proficiency
2. To determine motor proficiencies in specific subtest areas
3. To provide empirical data to meet criteria for placement of functional skill development
4. To determine relative areas of strengths and weaknesses in motor ability
5. To predict success in activity programs

Some professionals criticize the use of motor ability tests because the tests are not directly related to instructional goals and performance objectives. For example, a motor test may identify a child as being "deficient" in "gross body coordination," a so-called underlying motor ability, but the test does not link the result to a performance objective. The evaluator may well ask, "If Johnny is deficient in gross body coordination, what observable, measurable performance objectives are appropriate for Johnny that fit into the third-grade physical education curriculum?" Motor ability tests are recommended to be used with other validated tests of skills or functionally based curriculums that are consistent with the program goals for all children. For example, if all children should develop balance and object control skills by the third grade, the motor tests can be used in conjunction with peer evaluations at each grade level. Some commonly used motor ability tests follow.

The Bruininks-Oseretsky Test of Motor Proficiency (BOTMP)

The Bruininks-Oseretsky Test of Motor Proficiency (Bruininks, 1978) is a test of general motor proficiency for children 4½–14½ years of age (see Figure 6.2). An individually administered test, it assesses motor proficiency in gross motor and fine motor areas. The eight subtests include:

1. Running speed and agility: measure of speed during a shuttle run
2. Balance: measures static and dynamic balance
3. Bilateral coordination: test of sequential and simultaneous coordination of upper and lower limbs
4. Strength: measures arm-shoulder, abdominal, and leg strength
5. Upper-limb coordination: assesses coordination of visual tracking with arm and hand movements
6. Response speed: measures speed of response to a moving visual stimulus
7. Visual-motor control: assesses the coordination of precise hand and visual movement
8. Upper-limb speed and dexterity: measures hand and finger dexterity, hand and arm speed

The complete test battery provides three estimates of motor ability: a gross motor composite score, a fine motor composite score, and a general index of motor proficiency. For situations such as screening when a brief overview of motor ability is desired, the short form of the test, requiring approximately 20 minutes for administration, can be used.

The complete battery takes about one hour to administer to an individual. The manual has clearly written directions with illustrations to aid in administration. We recommend that the test be studied and administered by an appropriately trained professional. The test is relatively easy to score with guidelines for converting raw scores to percentiles and stanines, and age equivalent scores. The most valuable information provided by the test battery is comparative information about general motor proficiency relative to age group peers.

The Bruininks-Oseretsky Test of Motor Proficiency was standardized on a representative sample of 765 children from 4½–14½ years of age. It was one of the first

Complete Battery:

SUBTEST	POINT SCORE Maximum	Subject's	STANDARD SCORE Test Table 23	Composite Table 24	PERCENTILE RANK Table 25	STANINE Table 25	OTHER *Age (Equiv.)*
GROSS MOTOR-SUBTESTS							
1. Running Speed and Agility	15	8	21				7-8
2. Balance	32	16	13				5-2
3. Bilateral Coordination	20	9	23				7-11
4. Strength	42	5	11				4-11
GROSS MOTOR COMPOSITE.........			*68 sum	56	72	6	6-5
5. Upper-Limb Coordination	21	13	*21				6-11
FINE MOTOR SUBTESTS							
6. Response Speed	17	5	16				6-2
7. Visual-Motor Control	24	18	23				8-5
8. Upper-Limb Speed and Dexterity	72	27	20				6-8
FINE MOTOR COMPOSITE.........			*59 sum	64	92	8	6-8
BATTERY COMPOSITE.........			*148 sum	63	90	8	6-9

*To obtain Battery Composite Add Gross Motor Composite, Subtest 5 Standard Score, and Fine Motor Composite. Check result by adding Standard Scores on Subtests 1–8.

Short Form:

	POINT SCORE Maximum	Subject's	STANDARD SCORE Table 27	PERCENTILE RANK Table 27	STANINE Table 27
SHORT FORM	98				

FIGURE 6.2   Bruininks-Oseretsky Test of Motor Proficiency: Test Profile (or Score Summary)

motor tests to be developed from an excellent standardization program. Test-retest reliability coefficients are 87 percent for the long form and 86 percent for the short form. Validity data presented in the test manual are considered by Bruininks (1978, p. 28) as content and construct validity. These results support the use of the test to screen children for motor difficulties. General consensus is that the Bruininks is not a definitive assessment of motor development and has some limitations, but possesses potential for answering motor proficiency of children and identifying children with special needs (Gallahue, 1989). In addition, the Motor Skills Inventory (MSI) and the accompanying Motor Development Curriculum for Children developed by Werder and Bruininks (1988) can be used to give a criterion-based performance on a pass (+) or fail (–) basis. Bruininks-Oseretsky test scores can be used to predict performance on MSI test items. Werder and Bruininks (1988) indicated that the BOTMP can be administered at the beginning and end of a program with the MSI being administered more frequently throughout the year for periodic assessments of each skill to document progress.

Peabody Developmental Motor Scales (Folio and Fewell, 1983)

The Peabody Developmental Motor Scales (PDMS) were designed to assess fine and gross motor skills from birth to 7 years of age as shown in Figure 6.3 (Folio and Fewell, 1983). Like the Brigance, the skills are based on developmental landmarks

Name _Kimberly_	Date of Testing	Yr.	Mo.	Day
		1982	4	16
Educational Program _Rose Hill_	Date of Birth	1977	4	14
Examiner _J. Butler_	Chronological Age	5	0	2
Examination Center _Rose Hill_	Age in Months		60	

SUMMARY

	Gross Motor	Fine Motor
Basal Age Level	24-29	30-35
Ceiling Age Level	60-71	72-83
Scaled Score	552	564
Age Equivalent	42	52
Mean Motor Age Equivalent	= 48.5	

GROSS-MOTOR SCALE

	Raw Score	Percentile	z-score	Developmental Motor Quotient
Skill A — Reflexes	n	n	n	n
Skill B — Balance	55	05	-1.64	75
Skill C — Nonlocomotor	68	<02	-3.42	49
Skill D — Locomotor	80	<01	-5.49	18
Skill E — Receipt and Propulsion	37	04	-1.75	74
Total Score	264	<01	-4.16	38

FINE-MOTOR SCALE

	Raw Score	Percentile	z-score	Developmental Motor Quotient
Skill A — Grasping	43	02	-2.05	69
Skill B — Hand Use	n	n	n	n
Skill C — Eye-Hand Coordination	86	20	-.84	87
Skill D — Manual Dexterity	23	<02	<-2.05	<69
Total Score	204	03	-1.88	72

SCORING

GROSS MOTOR	Cumulative Basal Score		Sum Through Ceiling Age		Raw Score	Max. Score	Max. Age
Skill A	24	+	0	=	24★	24	8
Skill B	36	+	19	=	55		
Skill C	64	+	4	=	68		
Skill D	60	+	20	=	80		
Skill E	16	+	21	=	37		
Total Score		+		=	264		
FINE MOTOR	Cumulative Basal Score		Sum Through Ceiling Age		Raw Score	Max. Score	Max. Age
Skill A	21	+	22	=	43★	44	42
Skill B	48	+	4	=	52★	52	36
Skill C	60	+	26	=	86		
Skill D	14	+	9	=	23		
Total Score		+		=	204		

*Do not transfer to cover page if child is as old or older than age listed *and* obtains maximum score. Instead record ▷ (for normal) in the appropriate space on the front cover.

FIGURE 6.3   Kimberly's performance

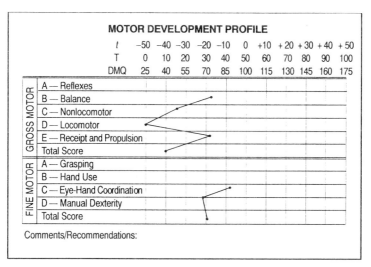

FIGURE 6.3—*Continued*

Copyright © 1983. Reproduced with permission of The Riverside Publishing Company, Chicago, Illinois.

and are scored on a pass-fail criteria of 0, 1, or 2. Zero indicates the child cannot or would not attempt the task, 1 indicates a clear resemblance to the criterion, and 2 is indicative of criterion-level performance. Standard scores—Z-scores, T-scores, and Developmental Motor Quotients (DMQ), can be obtained from raw scores. Folio and Fewell (1983) recommend using the DMQ and either Z-scores or T-scores (not both). This test is easy to use and has some utility in programming since it has an accompanying curriculum. The 282 PDMS items assessed include reflexes, balance, nonlocomotor, locomotor, and receipt and propulsion skills. The fine motor scale includes grasping, hand use, eye-hand coordination, and manual dexterity. Content validity is based on items of other validated motor development tests, while test-relevant reliability was reported as 95 percent for gross motor and 80 percent for fine motor skills.

Because this test is widely accepted in early intervention and is easy to use, we recommend consideration for use with infants and toddlers with disabilities. Folio and Fewell (1983) have indicated that the PDMS does not include norms for children with disabilities but provides vital information that is valid and useful in identifying development needs. The accompanying curriculum is helpful in early movement analysis. From personal observations and use in clinical and school-based settings, the Peabody and Brigance are two functional tests that provide useful information on motor development.

The Movement Assessment of Infants

The Movement Assessment of Infants (Chandler, Andrews, and Swanson, 1981) is viewed as a developmental tool with neuromotor implications. Since it is designed for birth to 1 year of age, the movement categories assessed include muscle tone, primitive reflexes, autonomic reactions, and volitional movement. Fewell (1991) indicated that it would be appropriate for developing a treatment plan but not for diagnosing or evaluating movement problems since it is concentrated during the first year.

Because of the limited scope (0–1 year) this assessment may not be beneficial for all children. It appears that early screening and intervention can be interpreted from neurological problems occurring during the first year. Information on the infant's early development would be extremely helpful when selecting appropriate developmental assessment tools and implementing intervention strategies.

Test of Gross Motor Development (TGMD)

The TGMD (Ulrich, 1985) is designed for assessment of children from 3–10 years of age in 12 gross motor patterns (see Table 6.2). The locomotor items include running, galloping, hopping, leaping, jumping, skipping, and sliding, while manipulative skills include striking, bouncing, catching, kicking, and throwing.

Measures of young children's primary motor patterns come in an easy to administer package with selected criteria for each skill. Test-retest reliability to 96 percent for the locomotor items and 97 percent for the manipulative items was reported. Content validity is reported from the evaluation of a panel of three judges concerning the appropriateness of test items for young children, while construct validity was established by factor analysis techniques.

Because this test is so straightforward and easy to administer, it is recommended for use in evaluating motor patterns in young children. For example, in catching there are four criteria:

1. Elbows flexed and hands in front of the body
2. Arms extended in preparation for ball contact
3. Ball is caught and controlled by the hands
4. Elbows bent to absorb force

The performance criteria are judged at 0 (absent) to 1 (present) to 2 if the objective is achieved. This instrument is helpful in identifying areas of motor weakness and in developing instructional programs.

Ohio State University Scale of Intra-Gross Motor Assessment (OSU-SIGMA)

The SIGMA (Loovis and Ersing, 1979) was designed to assess 11 motor skills in children 2½–14 years of age. It is a criterion-referenced instrument with four levels of development for each skill as to their ability at each level. As the level of the individual's development rises he or she should be able to progress to the next level of motor development. Motor skills included are walking, stair-climbing, running, throwing, catching, long-jumping, hopping, skipping, stretching, kicking, and ladder climbing. The test has some interesting components and is helpful in discriminating levels or maturing of patterns.

Movement Assessment Battery for Children (Movement ABC)

The Movement Assessment Battery for Children is a revised version of the Test of Motor Impairment (TOMI) that was designed to measure motor impairment in children from the ages of 4–12 (Henderson and Sudgen, 1992). The assessment has

TABLE 6.2 The Test of Gross Motor Development

TGMD

TEST OF GROSS MOTOR DEVELOPMENT

Name _____

School/Agency _____

Sex: Male _____ Female _____ Grade _____

Dale A. Ulrich

TESTING INFORMATION

1ST TESTING				2ND TESTING			
	Year	Month	Day		Year	Month	Day
Date Tested	_____	_____	_____	Date Tested	_____	_____	_____
Date of Birth	_____	_____	_____	Date of Birth	_____	_____	_____
Chronological Age	_____	_____	_____	Chronological Age	_____	_____	_____

Examiner's Name	Examiner's Name
Examiner's Title	Examiner's Title
Purpose of Testing	Purpose of Testing

RECORD OF SCORES

1ST TESTING

Subtests	Raw Scores	%iles	Std. Scores
Locomotor Skills	_____	_____	_____
Object Control Skills	_____	_____	_____

Sum of Standard Scores = _____

Gross Motor Development
Quotient (GMDQ) = _____

2ND TESTING

Subtests	Raw Scores	%iles	Std. Scores
Locomotor Skills	_____	_____	_____
Object Control Skills	_____	_____	_____

Sum of Standard Scores = _____

Gross Motor Development
Quotient (GMDQ) = _____

COMMENTS/RECOMMENDATIONS

_____

_____

_____

_____

TABLE 6.2—*Continued*

LOCOMOTOR SKILLS

Skill	Equipment	Directions	Performance Criteria	1st	2nd
RUN	50 feet of clear space, colored tape, chalk or other marking device	Mark off two lines 50 feet apart	1. Brief period where both feet are off the ground		
			2. Arms in opposition to legs, elbows bent		
		Instruct student to "run fast" from one line to the other	3. Foot placement near or on a line (not flat footed)		
			4. Nonsupport leg bent approximately 90 degrees (close to buttocks)		
GALLOP	A minimum of 30 feet of clear space	Mark off two lines 30 feet apart Tell student to gallop from one line to the other three times Tell student to gallop leading with one foot and then the other	1. A step forward with the lead foot followed by a step with the trailing foot to a position adjacent to or behind the lead foot		
			2. Brief period where both feet are off the ground		
			3. Arms bent and lifted to waist level		
			4. Able to lead with the right and left foot		
HOP	A minimum of 15 feet of clear space	Ask student to hop 3 times, first on one foot and then on the other	1. Foot of nonsupport leg is bent and carried in back of the body		
			2. Nonsupport leg swings in pendular fashion to produce force		
			3. Arms bent at elbows and swing forward on take off		
			4. Able to hop on the right and left foot		
LEAP	A minimum of 30 feet of clear space	Ask student to leap Tell him/her to take large steps leaping from one foot to the other	1. Take off on one foot and land on the opposite foot		
			2. A period where both feet are off the ground (longer than running)		
			3. Forward reach with arm opposite the lead foot		

TABLE 6.2—*Continued*

LOCOMOTOR SKILLS

Skill	Equipment	Directions	Performance Criteria	1st	2nd
HORIZONTAL JUMP	10 feet of clear space, tape or other marking devices	Mark off a starting line on the floor, mat, or carpet Have the student start behind the line Tell the student to "jump far"	1. Preparatory movement includes flexion of both knees with arms extended behind the body 2. Arms extend forcefully forward and upward, reaching full extension above head 3. Take off and land on both feet simultaneously 4. Arms are brought downward during landing		
SKIP	A minimum of 30 feet of clear space, marking device	Mark off two lines 30 feet apart Tell the student to skip from one line to the other three times	1. A rhythmical repetition of the step-hop on alternate feet 2. Foot of nonsupport leg carried near surface during hop 3. Arms alternately moving in opposition to legs at about waist level		
SLIDE	A minimum of 30 feet of clear space, colored tape or other marking device	Mark off two lines 30 feet apart Tell the student to slide from one line to the other three times facing the same direction	1. Body turned sideways to desired direction of travel 2. A step sideways followed by a slide of the trailing foot to a point next to the lead foot 3. A short period where both feet are off the floor 4. Able to slide to the right and to the left side		

LOCOMOTOR SKILLS SUBTEST SCORE

From Ulrich, D., *The Test of Gross Motor Development.* Used with permission of Pro-Ed, 1985.

two parts: an individually administered Performance Test requiring the child to perform a series of motor tasks, and a Checklist designed to be administered by a parent or teacher who is familiar with the child's functioning (Henderson and Sudgen, 1992). Groupings are categorized by the following age bands:

Age Band 1—5 and 6 years
Age Band 2—7 and 8 years
Age Band 3—9 and 10 years
Age Band 4—11 years and over

According to Henderson and Sudgen (1992), the Movement ABC is a comprehensive assessment that yields normative and qualitative measures of manual dexterity, ball skills, and balance (static and dynamic). Major categories include (a) items such as threading beads, training, piercing holes, cutouts, and other fine motor items, (b) ball skills, including throwing beanbags and balls, catching a bounced ball, catching off a wall with one hand, and hitting a target, and (c) static and dynamic balance items such as balance boards, beam walking, jumping over a cord, and clapping. Henderson and Sudgen (1992) indicated that requirements of the tasks in each level are identical but vary slightly for use with each age band. In addition, for each age band a qualitative observation is available to note variables such as concentration, confidence, posture, and control that relate to the child's behavior during testing.

Items are scored at the age level of the child, such as the number of seconds to complete a trial or number of catches executed out of ten attempts. If a child does not start a task, the score is recorded as a failed attempt (F), inappropriate (I) for a child, or refusal (R) to attempt a task. A shorter version (the Movement ABC Checklist) provides an opportunity to screen and monitor children on a daily basis and includes 48 questions in Sections 1–4 with responses from 0 (very well) to 3 (not close).

The following sections detail movement over what Henderson and Sudgen (1992, p. 25) refer to as more complex interactions:

Section 1   The child is stationary and the environment is stable.
Section 2   The child is moving and the environment is stable.
Section 3   The child is stationary and the environment is changing.
Section 4   The child is moving and the environment is changing.

Section 5 of the Checklist provides behavioral information that may influence performance and movement competence on Sections 1–4 (Henderson and Sudgen, 1992). For example, Section 5 is used to interpret or consider if the behavior will (1) prevent a child from demonstrating his or her time capability and (2) should the behavior be related to future management or remedial programs.

The first four sections are then scored to determine if children are "at risk" (15 percent of the population) or have definite movement problems (5 percent of the population). Behavior factors from Section 5 are ranked High, Medium, or Low as contributing factors to the child's performance.

Henderson and Sudgen (1992) indicate that once the Checklist is used to validate movement competence in a one-to-one setting, the Performance Test will provide a more detailed diagnostic procedure and aid in long-term planning. This revision of the previous Test of Motor Impairment (TOMI) provides a promising screening and diagnostic assessment procedure that can be used to compare children at various ages on motor skill performance, identify potential movement problems, and provide accurate information for program planning.

I CAN

The *I CAN* Program is not a test, but a curriculum that has a built-in assessment system (Kelly and Wessel, 1990). The *I CAN* Program is a task-analyzed, individualized physical education system that is a criterion-referenced measure of the current level of performance. The *I CAN* curriculum offers a set of diagnostic-prescriptive teaching resource materials with a curriculum structure designed for use with primary school children. It provides a system for training teachers in planning, assessing, prescribing, teaching, and evaluating student progress in physical education. The program is flexible enough for a variety of settings and is individualized. The instrument facilitates communication with parents and provides a management tool for teachers. *I CAN* addresses activities provided in the following skill areas:

1. Primary skills: fundamental skills, body management, health and fitness, aquatics
2. Secondary skills: backyard and neighborhood activities, team sports, outdoor activities, dance, and individual sports
3. Preschool skills: locomotor skills, object control skills, play equipment skills, body control skills, participation in play situation skills
4. Associated skills: self-concept, social skills

Scores on specific motor skill objectives are marked on a performance score sheet, which is also used to score progress on objectives. Skills are assessed in levels performed with assistance, without assistance, motive patterns, and/or distance, speed, or accuracy. Figure 6.4 shows a sample score sheet.

Advantages of *I CAN* and its criterion-referenced assessment are relevance and ability to track continuous progress. Disadvantages include lack of comparative test data (percentiles), lack of reliability and validity information, time required to assess each objective, and relatively high cost. It should also be noted that *I CAN* is based on task analyses of mature patterns of movement, so beginning or entry level components of the pattern may not be addressed. However, *I CAN* assessment is relevant to instructional and program planning on most motor and fitness skills of young children.

The *I CAN* preschool and primary skills assessment materials are most useful for elementary physical education teachers and for physical education teachers of children with mild to severe disabilities. The leisure and recreation assessment materials are most useful with secondary school individuals and adults with disabilities.

CLASS PERFORMANCE SCORE SHEET/PERFORMANCE OBJECTIVE OVERHAND THROW

I CAN SCORING

Assessment:
X = Achieved
O = Not Achieved

Reassessment:
Ⓧ = Achieved
Ø = Not Achieved

FOCAL POINTS

a Overhand Motion
  b Ball Release
    a Eyes on Target
      b Overhand Motion
        a Arm Exten/Side Orient
          b Weight Transfer
            c Hip and Spine Rotation
              d Follow Through
                e Smooth Integration
                  Angle of Release 45°
                    Accuracy

STD
10 ft. distance.
20 ft. target at 15 ft. 2/3 times
2/3 times
age/sex norm. 2/3 times
8 ft. target at 50 ft. 2/3 times

*PRIMARY RESPONSES
N — Nonattending
NR — No response
UR — Unrelated response
O — Other (specify in comments)

NAME	1 a	1 b	2 a	2 b	3 a	3 b	3 c	3 d	3 e	4	5	COMMENTS
1. John G.	Ⓧ	X	Ⓧ	Ⓧ	O	Ⓧ	Ⓧ	O	O	O	O	Throws side arm
2. Katie	X	X	X	X	Ⓧ	Ⓧ	Ⓧ	X	O	O	O	
3. Susan	X	X	X	X	X	X	X	X	X	X	O	Practice accuracy
4. Mark	X	X	X	X	O	X	O	Ⓧ	O	O	O	Faces target
5. John S.	X	X	X	X	X	X	X	Ⓧ	O	O	O	Follow through inconsistent
6. Scott	Ⓧ	X	O	Ⓧ	O	O	O	O	O	O	O	Throws underhand
7. Judy	X	X	O	X	O	O	O	O	O	O	O	Doesn't look at target
8. Cindy	X	X	X	X	Ⓧ	X	Ⓧ	X	O	O	O	Faces target
9. Kirk	X	X	X	X	X	X	X	X	O	O	O	Jerky
10. Joanie	X	X	X	X	X	X	Ⓧ	X	O	O	O	
11. Larry	X	X	X	X	Ⓧ	X	X	X	O	O	O	Arm bent
12. Chuck	X	X	Ⓧ	Ⓧ	O	Ⓧ	O	O	O	O	O	Throws underhand or side arm unless assisted
13. Linda	X	X	X	X	X	X	X	X	Ⓧ	Ⓧ	O	nearly mature
14. Sherry	X	X	X	X	Ⓧ	X	Ⓧ	X	Ⓧ	O	O	Inconsistent beginning position
15. Greg	X	X	X	X	X	X	X	X	Ⓧ	Ⓧ	Ⓧ	nearly mature

FIGURE 6.4 *I CAN* score sheet

From Wessel, J.A., Director, *I CAN Primary Skills.* Used with permission of Pro-Ed.

Basic Gross Motor Assessment

Although classified a gross motor assessment and not considered by the author as a perceptual motor test, the Basic Gross Motor Assessment contains many measures of perceptual motor functioning (Hughes, 1979). Subtests include: (a) static balance with a stork stand, (b) stride jump, (c) heel-toe walk for dynamic balance, (d) hopping, (e) skipping, (f) target toss with bean bags, (g) object control with a yo-yo, and (h) ball handling (e.g., catching, throwing, dribbling) with a 7-inch ball. The scoring system of 0–3 is as follows:

    3—no difficulty

    2—1 observed difficulty

1—3 observed difficulties

0—unable to perform 3 observed difficulties

Content validity was reported by a panel of six authorities while construct validity was reported by factor analysis. Test-retest reliability was 97 percent and internal consistency was 71 percent.

Perceptual Motor Tests

Interrelated with motor development is perceptual motor functioning and how it contributes to or detracts from motor development or skill performance. For example, the modalities of hearing, vision, touch, and kinesthetic awareness are all important facilitators of motor proficiency. Deficits in perceptual functioning may contribute to delayed development. For example, an individual with a visual impairment cannot use visual perception to imitate or refine movements. However, he or she may use other perceptual modalities. Likewise, some individuals may have sight, yet they may not be able to interpret visual input and, therefore, remain unable to formulate an effective motor response.

Salvia and Ysseldyke (1991) indicated that assessing perception is vital to identifying difficulties that interfere with learning as well as brain injury. A critical concern is that functioning is affected by perception, and assessment of perception is important in determining the overall capabilities of the individual. In addition, perception should be specific to the modality or stage being assessed. Visual perception differs from assessing auditory or tactile perception. Likewise, when using an information processing model of: (1) input, (2) decision making, (3) output, and (4) a feedback loop, it becomes essential to recognize the stage at which perception is occurring or not functioning. Several assessments which may be helpful in this process follow.

The Purdue Perceptual-Motor Survey (PPMS)

The Purdue Perceptual-Motor Survey (Roach and Kephart, 1966, p. 2) was designed to assess "qualitatively the perceptual-motor abilities of children in the early grades." The test measures perceptual-motor performance in five areas: balance and posture, body image and differentiation, ocular control, form perception, and perceptual-motor matching. These areas include a total of 22 scoreable items. Roach and Kephart (1966, p. 11) stated that the test was not designed to diagnose, but "to allow the clinician to observe perceptual-motor behavior in a series of behavioral performances."

The survey is designed to be administered individually to children, ages 6–10, who do not have specific sensory or physical disabilities (e.g., blindness, paralysis, or physical impairments). Behaviors sampled in the five areas include the following:

1. Balance and posture: walking a balance beam and jumping
2. Body image and differentiation: identification of body parts, imitation of movement, obstacle course, Kraus-Weber, and "angels in the snow"
3. Perceptual-motor match: drawing a circle, drawing two circles simultaneously, drawing a lateral line, and drawing two straight vertical lines simultaneously

4. Ocular control: movement of eyes following a flashlight, and convergence on objects
5. Form perception: copying seven geometric forms

The scoring procedures are primarily qualitative and subjective. The form is essentially a checklist that enables the scorer to note specific difficulties on each item.

The Purdue Perceptual-Motor Survey was standardized on 200 children, aged 6–10, who were known to be free of motor difficulties. The authors report a test-retest reliability of 95 percent, based on scores of 30 children from the standardization sample. We have little valid information that the survey tests what it purports to measure. The instrument should be used cautiously and be supplemented with other physical education performance information.

Perceptual-Motor Screening Checklist

The Perceptual-Motor Screening Checklist provides an overall screening for determining potential perceptual problems. Sherrill (1976) indicated that individuals with more than ten checked items should be referred for more intensive observation. Sherrill also recommends the Sherrill Perceptual-Motor Tasks for Physical Education (1993) testing and teaching criterion-referenced instrument that includes: (1) identification of body parts, (2) right-left discriminations, (3) changing positions, (4) crossing the midline, (5) imitation of movements, (6) imitation of sports movements, (7) visual tracking, (8) static balance, (9) dynamic balance, and (10) lateral dominance.

Developmental Test of Visual Perception (DTVP-2)

The DTVP-2 is a revision of Frostig's original Test of Visual Perception. The DTVP-2 includes eight subtests: Eye-Hand Coordination, Copying, Spatial Relations, Position in Space, Figure-Ground, Visual Closure, Visual-Motor Speed, and Form Constancy (see Figure 6.5). Hammill et al. (1993) indicated that the DTVP-2 is based on updated theories of visual perception and is suitable for children aged 4–9 years providing scores for pure visual perception (without motor response) and visual motor integration. The DTVP-2 was standardized on approximately 2,000 children and reports internal consistency and stability reliability scores 80 percent and above for all ages. Criterion validity was established by correlating items with the Bender Visual Motor Gestalt Test, the Developmental Test of Visual-Motor Integration (VMI) and the Motor-Free Visual Perception Test (MVPT). Hammill et al. (1993) also reported construct validity from correlations with tests of mental ability, achievement, and age.

Southern California Perceptual-Motor Test (SCPMT)

The SCPMT is designed to measure sensory integration in children 4–8 years of age (Ayres, 1980). Six subtests include imitation of postures, crossing the midline, bilateral motor coordination, right-left discriminations, standing balance—eyes open, and standing balance—eyes closed. This test is extremely difficult to administer and emphasizes training from an occupational therapist before administration. The use of this instrument is not recommended with the information provided in other tests.

DTVP-2

**Developmental Test
of Visual Perception**
Second Edition

**PROFILE/EXAMINER
RECORD FORM**

Section I. Identifying Information

Name: _Sarah Boston_   Male ___ Female ✓

	Year	Month	Day
Date Tested	92	11	16
Date of Birth	85	7	8
Age	7	4	8

Examiner's name: _____
Examiner's title: _____
School: _Covert Avenue School_   Grade _2_

Section II. Record of DTPV-2 Subtest and Composite Scores

Subtest	Raw Score	Age Equiv.	%ile	GVP	MRP	VMI	Composite	Quotients	%iles	Age Equiv.
1. Eye-Hand Coordination	140	5-10	25	8		8	General Visual Perception	103	58	7-6
2. Position in Space	17	6-3	37	9	9					
3. Copying	23	7-3	50	10		10				
4. Figure-Ground	14	10-7	75	12	12		Motor-Reduced Visual Perception	102	55	7-0
5. Spatial Relations	40	9-7	84	13		13				
6. Visual Closure	12	7-10	63	11	11					
7. Visual-Motor Speed	13	8-2	63	11		+ 11	Visual-Motor Integration	103	58	7-8
8. Form Constancy	10	5-7	37	+ 9	+ 9					

Subtest Standard Scores Sum = [83] [41] [42]

Section III. Profile of Test Scores

	Subtest Scores									Composite Scores				Other Test Scores						

Std. Scores	Eye-Hand Coordination	Position in Space	Copying	Figure-Ground	Spatial Relations	Visual Closure	Visual-Motor Speed	Form Constancy	Std. Scores	Quotients	General Visual Perception	Motor-Reduced Visual Perception	Visual-Motor Integration	1	2	3	4	5	6	7	Quotients
20	·	·	·	·	·	·	·	·	20	150	·	·	·	·	·	·	·	·	·	·	150
19	·	·	·	·	·	·	·	·	19	145	·	·	·	·	·	·	·	·	·	·	145
18	·	·	·	·	·	·	·	·	18	140	·	·	·	·	·	·	·	·	·	·	140
17	·	·	·	·	·	·	·	·	17	135	·	·	·	·	·	·	·	·	·	·	135
16	·	·	·	·	·	·	·	·	16	130	·	·	·	·	·	·	·	·	·	·	130
15	·	·	·	·	·	·	·	·	15	125	·	·	·	·	·	·	·	·	·	·	125
14	·	·	·	·	·	·	·	·	14	120	·	·	·	·	·	·	·	·	·	·	120
13	·	·	·	·	X	·	·	·	13	115	·	·	·	·	X	·	·	·	·	·	115
12	·	·	·	X	·	·	·	·	12	110	·	·	·	X	·	·	·	·	·	·	110
11	·	·	·	·	·	X	X	·	11	105	X	·	X	·	·	·	·	·	·	·	105
10	·	·	X	·	·	·	·	·	10	100	·	X	·	·	·	·	·	·	·	·	100
9	X	·	·	·	·	·	·	X	9	95	·	·	·	·	·	·	·	·	·	·	95
8	X	·	·	·	·	·	·	·	8	90	·	·	·	·	·	·	·	·	·	·	90
7	·	·	·	·	·	·	·	·	7	85	·	·	·	·	·	·	·	·	·	·	85
6	·	·	·	·	·	·	·	·	6	80	·	·	·	·	·	·	·	·	·	·	80
5	·	·	·	·	·	·	·	·	5	75	·	·	·	·	·	·	·	·	·	·	75
4	·	·	·	·	·	·	·	·	4	70	·	·	·	·	·	·	·	·	·	·	70
3	·	·	·	·	·	·	—	·	3	65	·	·	·	·	·	·	·	·	·	·	65
2	·	·	·	·	·	·	·	·	2	60	·	·	·	·	·	·	·	·	·	·	60
1	·	·	·	·	·	·	·	·	1	55	·	·	·	·	·	·	·	·	·	·	55

FIGURE 6.5   Example of a Completed Profile/Examiner Record Form

Copyright © 1993. Used with permission of Pro-Ed.

Other Perceptual Components

Other perceptual components can also be assessed to determine various problems encountered by children. Many are available in perceptual motor tests, while others may be specific to deficiencies required to develop and initiate a program plan. Most can be used in a checklist to note the presence or absence of the movement.

Spatial Relations—the inability to perceive the relationship of an object in space to another or to the person. Crossing the midline is a spatial relations phenomenon, as is putting movements in the right order (e.g., positioning the arms, legs or trunk in relation to executing a movement). Test questions may involve standing next to the teacher/leader, moving to the other side of the gymnasium or playground, crossing the midline using a bat that can be grasped with two hands, or throwing a ball or skipping.

Form Constancy—the ability to detect differences in form and shape, such as between a football and basketball, or, in contrast, identifying the object if the object is placed in various positions such as upside down, left, or right. Tactile, visual, and verbal information should be used to initiate movements.

Position in Space—the ability to perceive laterality or directionality when objects are placed in different positions in relation to the child (e.g., balls or other objects in various locations). Fitness or motor assessments may require lifting the arms above the head or the foot from a balance beam.

Depth Perception—the distance perception occurs when climbing stairs, overshooting or undershooting while reaching for an object, or misjudging a step or a curb. Difficulties may require compensation techniques or use of other sensory modalities to provide correct information.

Vertical disorientation may also affect motor performance, especially in posture and gait, since everything seems tilted or distorted. Moving through the environment may be distorted if the individual does not compensate.

Agnosias—the inability to recognize familiar objects in one modality while recognizing the object through another modality. Modalities may be intact yet not functioning due to interruption of the transmission of the sensory input. Common agnosia include visual, auditory, or tactile. Assessments can be implemented by identifying objects, such as a basketball, by touching or bouncing the ball, or in the case of auditory agnosia, identifying sounds with the eyes closed.

Apraxia—the inability to perform purposeful movements, although functional strength, attention, and coordination may be appropriate. Generally, apraxia is the result of dominant hemisphere lesions and may be associated with language difficulties or aphasia. The corresponding dysfunction in the motor domain disrupts skilled movements and motor planning required for movement execution. Initiation of postures and limb movements are common techniques in the assessment of apraxia.

Body Schema—the awareness of body parts and their functions. Parietal and temporal lobe dysfunctions may interfere with performing appropriate movement sequences on one side or from the opposite side. Initiation of movement sequences should be utilized, as well as statements concerning body awareness (e.g., placing hands above the head or below the waist).

Right-left discrimination difficulties may also be evident if the individual cannot execute movements when given commands for a specific direction. For example, the individual may be asked to point to specific body parts (e.g., touch your left ear, right foot) or to identify body parts from a visual model (e.g., poster) of a person.

References

Ayres, A. J. *Southern California Sensory Integration Tests.* Los Angeles: Western Psychological Services, 1980.

Bayley, N. A. *Manual for the Bayley Scales of Infant Development.* New York: The Psychological Corporation, 1993.

Brigance, A. *Brigance Diagnostic Inventory of Early Development.* North Billerica, MA: Curriculum Associates, 1978.

Bruininks, R. H. *Bruininks-Oseretsky Test of Motor Proficiency.* Circle Pines, MN: American Guidance Service, 1978.

Buros, O. K., Ed. *The Eighth Annual Mental Measurements Yearbook* (Vols. 1 and 2). Highland Park, NJ: Gryphon Press, 1985.

Capute, A. J., F. B. Palmer, B. F. Shapiro, R. C. Wachtel, A. Ross, and P. J. Accardo. *Primitive Reflex Profile.* Baltimore: University Park Press, 1984.

Chandler, L., M. Andrews, and M. Swanson. *The Movement Assessment of Infants.* Rolling Bay, WA: Infant Movement Research, 1981.

Fewell, R. "Trends in the Assessment of Infants and Toddlers with Disabilities." *Exceptional Children,* 58(2), 1991, 166–173.

Florentino, M. *Normal and Abnormal Development: The Influence of Primitive Reflexes on Motor Development.* Springfield, IL: Charles C Thomas, 1972.

Folio, M. R., and R. Fewell. *Peabody Developmental Motor Scales.* Allen, TX: DLM Teaching Resources, 1983.

Frankenburg, W. K., J. Dodds, and P. Archer. *Denver II (Technical Manual).* Denver: Denver Developmental Materials, Inc., 1990.

Frankenburg, W. K., J. Dodds, P. Archer, H. Shapiro, and B. Bresnick. "The Denver II: A Major Revision and Restandardization of the Denver Developmental Screening Test." *Pediatrics, 89*(1), 1992, 91, 97.

Frankenburg, W. K., A. Goldstein, and B. Camp. *The Revised Denver Developmental Screening Test, Reference Manual,* rev. ed. Denver, CO: LADOCA Project Publishing Foundation, 1975.

Gallahue, D. *Understanding Motor Development in Infants, Children and Adolescents.* Indianapolis: Benchmark Press, 1989.

Gesell, A., and C. S. Amatruda. *Gesell Developmental Schedules.* New York: Psychological Company, 1949.

Hammill, D. V., N. A. Pearson, and J. K. Voress. *Developmental Test of Visual Perception,* 2nd ed. Austin, TX: Pro-Ed, 1993.

Haywood, R. M. *Life Span Motor Development,* 2nd ed. Champaign, IL: Human Kinetics Publishers, 1993.

Henderson, S., and D. Sudgen. *Movement Assessment Battery for Children.* San Antonio, TX. Psychological Corporation, Harcourt Brace Jovanovich, 1992.

Herkowitz, J. "Assessing the Motor Development of Children: Presentation and Critique of Tests." M. Ridenour, Ed. *Motor Development.* Princeton, NJ: Princeton Book Company, 1978.

Horvat, M. *Physical Education and Sports for Exceptional Students.* Dubuque, IA: Wm. C. Brown, 1990.

Hughes, J. *Hughes Basic Gross Motor Assessment Manual.* Yonkers, NY: G.E. Miller, Inc., 1979.

Kelly, L., and J.A. Wessel. *I CAN: Primary Skills.* Austin, TX: Pro-Ed, 1990.

Loovis, M., and W.F. Ersing. Ohio State University SIGMA. *Assessing and Programming Gross Motor Development for Children.* Cleveland Heights, OH: Ohio Motor Assessment Associates, 1979.

McCarthy, D. *McCarthy Scales of Children's Abilities.* San Antonio, TX: The Psychological Corporation, 1972.

McCarthy, D. *McCarthy Screening Test.* San Antonio, TX: The Psychological Corporation, 1978.

McClenaghan, B., and D. Gallahue. *Fundamental Movement.* Philadelphia: W.B. Saunders, 1978.

Milani-Comparetti, A., and E.A. Gidoni. "A Pattern Analysis of Motor Development and its Disorders." *Developmental Medicine and Child Neurology, 11*, 1967, 625–630.

O'Sullivan, S.B., and T.J. Schmitz. *Physical Rehabilitation: Assessment and Treatment,* 2nd ed. Philadelphia: F.A. Davis Co., 1988.

Payne, G., and L. Issacs. *Human Motor Development: A Lifespan Approach,* 3rd ed. Mountain View, CA: Mayfield Publishers, 1995.

Roach, E.F., and N.C. Kephart. *The Purdue Perceptual-Motor Survey.* Columbus, OH: Charles E. Merrill, 1966.

Salvia, J., and J. Ysseldyke. *Assessment in Special and Remedial Education,* 4th ed. Boston: Houghton Mifflin, 1991.

Sanford, A. *The Learning Accomplishment Profile.* Winston-Salem, NC: Kaplan School Supply, 1975.

Sherrill, C. *Adapted Physical Education and Recreation,* 4th ed. Dubuque, IA: Wm. C. Brown, 1993.

Sherrill, C. Sherrill "Perceptual-Motor Screening Checklist." C. Sherrill, *Adapted Physical Education and Recreation.* Dubuque, IA: Wm. C. Brown, 1976.

Ulrich, D. *The Test of Gross Motor Development.* Austin, TX: Pro-Ed, 1985.

Werder, J., and R.H. Bruininks. *A Motor Development Curriculum for Children.* Circle Pines, MN: American Guidance Services, 1988.

Werder, J.K., and L.H. Kalakian. *Assessment in Adapted Physical Education.* Minneapolis: Burgess Publishing Co., 1985.

Wickstrom, R. *Fundamental Motor Patterns,* 3rd ed. Philadelphia: Lea and Febiger, 1983.

CHAPTER 7

Physical Fitness

Among the major goals of physical education and recreation, including adapted physical education and therapeutic recreation, are facilitating among all individuals the ability and desire to lead physically active, healthy lifestyles, and emphasizing the importance of fitness for many tasks that impact functional development and that are needed in community and work-related settings. Clearly, fitness is a great facilitator of these goals. One could argue that fitness is *the* great facilitator of enjoying activity and increasing the functional capabilities of individuals with disabilities. Given that fitness makes activity enjoyable and translates to community and work productivity, achieving, maintaining, and even improving fitness through activity should become a life-long reality and a functional component of the adapted physical education and therapeutic recreation programs. Adequate assessments should be utilized to determine specific levels of fitness and the effects of intervention programs designed to develop and maintain physical fitness.

In this chapter, fitness is defined and discussed according to its mutually exclusive components. A representative sample of fitness tests and test batteries will be presented.

Fitness among Individuals with Disabilities

Caution should always be used in making generalizations about persons with disabilities. Any generalizations, including fitness generalizations, about individuals with disabilities is fraught with potential pitfalls. From this perspective, the authors proceed advisedly and with caution.

The authors assert that individuals with disabilities, *as a group*, typically do not manifest fitness levels characteristic of their able-bodied counterparts. Historically, many factors have mitigated against individuals with disabilities achieving optimal, and, sometimes even minimal, fitness levels.

Often, a major factor limiting achievement of fitness potential among individuals with disabilities is underexpectations on the part of significant others. Underexpectations lead to underachievement when those holding underexpectations are, to name a few, parents, guardians, friends, peers, teachers, therapists, paraprofessionals, counselors, and program administrators. A greater dilemma is encountered when the significant others' underexpectations are but a microcosm of underexpectations held by society at large. In effect, underexpectations can be taught consciously or subconsciously by those listed above, and learned by individuals with disabilities.

To the extent that individuals with disabilities comprehend that others perceive them as being limited, low self-esteem may result. Perhaps one of the most viable avenues to improved self-esteem is maintaining parameters of fitness that promote a positive, healthy, active lifestyle. Being fit means being active, and being active is positive, healthy, and generalizes to effective integration in community settings. The net result can be a sense of feeling good about oneself that promotes positive self-esteem and self-assessment. Further, fitness that promotes an active lifestyle sends concrete "can do" messages to a society that sometimes regards individuals with disabilities from perspectives of what they "cannot do."

Fitness Defined

To adequately define the components of physical fitness is difficult, since many definitions of fitness abound and experts do not always agree. While there is widespread consensus that fitness is important (and, therefore, should be assessed), there is something less than consensus regarding the constellation of components that comprise fitness.

Historically, fitness components have been divided into two major categories, *physical* (i.e., health-related) *fitness* and *performance* or *motor fitness*. In recent years, interest in fitness, specifically labeled *health-related*, has enjoyed increased attention. Health-related fitness addresses fitness attributes that, according to Pate and Shepherd (1989), specifically facilitate day-to-day function and health maintenance. Health-related fitness components include the following (AAHPERD, 1988):

1. Muscular strength/endurance
2. Flexibility
3. Cardiorespiratory endurance (AAHPERD substitutes *aerobic* for *cardiorespiratory*)
4. Body composition

Health-related fitness is the major focus of this chapter (elements of motor fitness, such as balance, are included in Chapter 6). Power, because it results from a combination of strength and speed, will also be included in this chapter. Malina and Bouchard (1991) commonly use the terms explosive strength or power synonymously to describe the muscles' ability to exert maximal force in the shortest possible time (p. 188). Examples of specific health-related fitness tests that are laboratory-based, field-based, or used in each setting are included in Table 7.1.

Multidimensionality of Fitness: Implications for Selecting Test Items

In accepting the premise that fitness is multidimensional or is required in many developmental, performance, or work-related tasks, one accepts that the various components of physical fitness tend to exist mutually exclusive of one another. This mutual exclusivity phenomenon requires that different test items (i.e., items representative of each proficiency) be administered to ensure that performance with respect to each proficiency is, in fact, measured. Further, when measuring proficiency with respect to any given component, more than one test item likely will be necessary to ensure that proficiency with respect to that given component has been thoroughly addressed. For example, when measuring strength, arm strength will not necessarily be predictive of trunk or leg strength. For the sake of thoroughness, specific strength test items should be administered to make valid assessments of strength in each specific muscle group deemed important. Given that the components of fitness tend to exist mutually exclusive of one another, each component deemed important should be addressed separately.

Components of Fitness

Muscular Strength and Endurance

Muscular strength and muscular endurance are separate fitness entities and are major considerations for increasing the functional capabilities of individuals with disabilities. Strength and endurance are essential components of fitness that correlate highly with self-sufficiency, job performance, and work productivity (Croce and Horvat, 1992; Nordgren and Backstrom, 1972; Shepherd, 1990). However, the line between strength and endurance often blurs, due in part to the ways by which these proficiencies are often measured. *Strength* is defined as maximal muscular exertion of relatively brief duration. Ideally, strength should be measured by the amount of force one can exert in a single, maximal effort. *Muscular endurance* is defined as submaximal exertion that extends over a relatively long period of time. Where strength involves brief, all-out effort, muscular endurance involves submaximal, extended effort. Since individuals with disabilities are typically required to rely on physical skills in the workplace, enhanced physical capabilities can make a significant contribution to overall vocational and social development (Tomporowski and Hayden, 1990). Therefore, it is imperative that professionals are able to accurately and reliably ascertain the functional strength of these individuals.

There are currently several methods for assessing the strength and endurance performance of individuals with disabilities. In laboratory settings, cable tensiometers, free weights, and isokinetic devices can be used to assess muscular strength. However, these tests are impractical to use either in field-based settings or when a large number of subjects must be tested in a short time period (see Table 7.1).

In order to accommodate these situations, more economical and practical assessment tests must often be employed. For example, upper extremity assessments in field-based settings commonly use push-ups, pull-ups and/or some modification

TABLE 7.1 Fitness Components and Appropriate Tests by Setting

Fitness Components	Laboratory	Combination	Field-Based
Muscular strength/endurance	Isokinetic dynamometer (Cybex, Kin-Com) Cable tensiometer (Baumgartner and Jackson, 1995)	Isotonic 1RM bench press, curls, lap pull-down (Fleck and Kraemer, 1993) 50% of 6RM to fatigue (Fleck and Kraemer, 1993) Manual muscle testers (Horvat et al., 1992, 1993) Hand grip dynamometer (Lafayette Instruments)	Pull-ups (AAHPERD, 1988) Modified pull-ups (Baumgartner, 1978) Flexed arm hang (FITNESSGRAM, 1992) Sit-ups (AAHPERD, 1988) Isometric push-up (Johnson and Lavay, 1988)
Flexibility	Leighton flexometer (Leighton, 1955)	Goniometer (Norkin and White, 1988) Length of muscle groups (Kendall, McCreary, and Provance, 1993)	Sit-and-reach (AAHPERD, 1988) Modified sit-and-reach (Hoeger et al., 1990)

Body composition	Underwater weighing (Malina and Bouchard, 1991) Potassium whole body counting (Malina and Bouchard, 1991) Bioelectrical impedance (Malina and Bouchard, 1991) Computerized tomography (Malina and Bouchard, 1991) Magnetic resonance (Malina and Bouchard, 1991) Anthropometry (Malina and Bouchard, 1991)	Skinfolds (FITNESSGRAM, 1992; Lohmann, 1987; AAHPERD, 1988)	Body mass index (Golding, Myers, and Sinning, 1989; AAHPERD, 1988) Girth measurements (Burgener, 1992)
Cardiorespiratory endurance	$\dot{V}O_2$ max treadmill (ACSM, 1980) $\dot{V}O_2$ max cycle ergometer (ACSM, 1980) $\dot{V}O_2$ max arm crank ergometer (ACSM, 1980) $\dot{V}O_2$ max Schwinn Air-Dyne (Pitetti and Tan, 1990)	PWC 170 (Bar-Or, 1983)	9 min or 12 min run for distance (AAHPERD, 1976) 1.5 mile run/walk (AAHPERD, 1988) 1.5 mile run/walk (AAHPERD, 1976) 20 min steady-state jog (FYT, 1980) 20 min shuttle run (Montgomery et al., 1992) Step test—pulse recovery (Reid, 1985) Rockport walking test (Kline et al., 1987)
Explosive strength/power	Vertisonic (Lafayette Instruments)	Wingate peak power test (Bar-Or, 1993) Margaria/Kalaman leg power test (Mathews and Fox, 1971)	Vertical jump (Clarke and Clarke, 1987) Long jump (Clarke and Clarke, 1987) Sargents jump (Sargent, 1921) Shot-put/medicine ball throw (McCloy and Young, 1954)

of these tests. When measuring the strength and endurance of the lower extremities, the most commonly used field-based tests are the long jump and vertical jump. Although some individuals consider these tests to be measures of power (Baumgartner and Jackson, 1995) each of these field-based tests is considered a relative measure of strength (Pate and Shepherd, 1989).

In children and individuals with disabilities, strength and endurance measures, such as the pull-up, often result in zero scores or, at best, inaccurate indicators of actual strength and/or functional capability. Body size and weight can also restrict or strongly influence physical performance (Shepherd, 1990). To offset these problems, researchers have attempted to minimize the effect of body weight and to eliminate zero scores that occur with upper body measures by developing modified pull-up tests or through the use of the flexed arm hang (Woods, Pate, and Burgess, 1992).

Field-based tests are widely variable in comparing children and individuals with disabilities. Variations based on levels of strength, body structure, and the rate and extent of growth at various developmental stages are evident (Woods et al., 1992). Most of these tests are not specific enough to isolate individual muscles; instead they test groups of muscles that work synergistically (Horvat, Croce, and Roswal, 1993).

Typically, muscular strength and endurance have been measured in practical settings using items including, but not limited to, pull-ups, sit-ups, push-ups, flexed arm hang, and parallel bar dips. A major problem encountered in utilizing such items is that the relative fitness level of the individual with the disability determines whether strength or endurance is being measured. If strength is, indeed, best measured by a single, maximal effort, then multiple repetition test items similar to those cited above are of questionable validity as strength measures. An individual able to execute, for example, only one pull-up would be demonstrating strength (albeit limited) in specific arm and shoulder girdle muscles. A child/client able to execute numerous repetitions of pull-ups would be demonstrating muscular endurance. As a rule of thumb, when the task's difficulty limits repetitions to ten or less, strength tends to be measured. Repetitions beyond ten begin to measure muscular endurance. According to Corbin and Lindsey (1994, p. 99) ". . . progressive resistance exercise using a maximum load (resistance) for three to ten repetitions in one to three sets three or four times per week will develop strength." One may infer from this premise that if three to ten repetitions maximum of any given activity develops strength, then three to ten repetitions of that activity, if the effort is maximal, also measures strength.

Strength can be measured more purely (according to the definition cited above) by using one or more of a number of devices that measure force exerted in terms of pounds or kilograms. In other settings, the use of 1 repetition max (1RM) on a universal gym, bench press, forearm curl, or latissimus dorsi pull-down can be determined and converted to a composite strength score. Furthermore, endurance tests using 50 percent of the individual's 1RM values (Berger, 1970) or 50 percent of 6RM max for younger children can also be used to provide a composite endurance score for the total number of repetitions (Kraemer and Fleck, 1993). The dilemma encountered here is that such devices often are not available in practical settings. Examples of such devices include spring scales, cable tensiometers, hand-grip dynamometers, and back and leg dynamometers (see Figures 7.1 through 7.3). These devices offer the advantage of enabling measurement of single, all-out efforts.

When interpreting strength measures, a factor to consider is the force exerted by the individual in relation to her or his body weight. For example, if a 125-pound person applied a given amount of leg strength force to a leg dynamometer, and another person weighing 100 pounds were to apply the same force, the second person would be judged the stronger. When assessing strength, one must often look beyond raw strength. One should interpret strength measures in terms of *strength per pound of body weight.* The importance of interpreting strength in terms of strength per pound of body weight is underscored by Rarick and Dobbins (1975). These investigators have determined that among the various fitness components, the component muscular strength correlates most highly with motor skill in children.

Strength can be measured (and developed) isotonically, isokinetically, and isometrically. When measuring isometric strength, it is important to ensure that repeated measures of the same individual or between individuals occur at precisely the same point (i.e., degree of angle at the joint) in each individual's range of

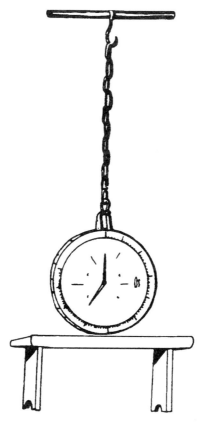

FIGURE 7.1 Back and leg (spring scale) dynamometer

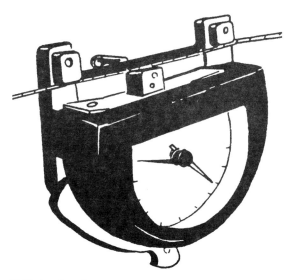

FIGURE 7.2   Cable tensiometer

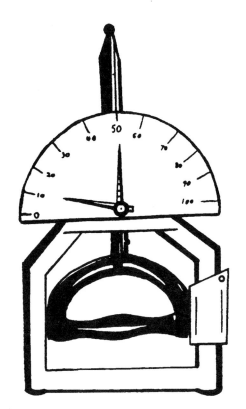

FIGURE 7.3   Grip dynamometer

motion. This is critical because strength within the same muscle or muscle group differs, often dramatically, when measured at different points throughout the muscle or muscle group's range of motion. When measuring strength isotonically or isokinetically, it is critical that individuals repeatedly exert force through the same range of motion. Typically, the best standardization procedure, unless other considerations preexist, is to have each person exert force through his or her entire range of motion. Getting an individual with a disability to exert force through an entire range, particularly with fatigue, lack of motivation and attention, is sometimes difficult. For validity's sake, only correctly performed repetitions can be counted.

Depending upon the individual's fitness level, items like sit-ups, push-ups, and flexed arm hang often will provide better measures of muscular endurance than strength. This is particularly true when items such as those above require substantially less than a single all-out effort. Repetitions of any given item as a measure of muscular endurance can be scored in two ways. A test item can require an individual to execute as many repetitions of a given activity as possible, or an item can determine how many repetitions can be performed within some given time limit. Each procedure has advantages and disadvantages. Items requiring maximum repetitions without regard to time may more validly measure endurance, although they may not be time effective. Items with time limitations, while they may increase time effectiveness, may introduce the unwanted element of muscle contraction speed or skill which, in turn, could contaminate a score believed to represent only endurance.

Flexibility

Flexibility is defined as "the ability to move the body and its parts through a wide range of motion without undue strain on the articulations and muscle attachments" (Johnson and Nelson, 1986). Inflexibility can heighten the likelihood of strain not only at attachment cites, but in the muscle belly itself.

When measuring flexibility, there is a need to recognize each individual's threshold of discomfort. Perception of discomfort is, of course, very subjective and unique to each individual. However, assessor sensitivity to each person's perception of discomfort is important to ensure that flexibility testing does not, in itself, put the individual at undue risk for incurring muscle strain. Recognizing the individual's level of discomfort is particularly critical if the person being tested is limited by muscle disease. For example, an individual with Duchenne muscular dystrophy may be more susceptible to muscle strain during testing than would a peer whose relative inflexibility is not necessarily a function of underlying muscle disease.

Concern for flexibility is important for a variety of reasons. Significant inflexibility places the person at risk of incurring muscle strain even while carrying out common, everyday tasks. Simply reaching for an item on the top shelf of a cupboard may produce muscle strain in some unfit individuals. Given this level of inflexibility and the attendant discomfort coming from trying to meet routine movement needs, the inflexible person's response often is to adopt a sedentary lifestyle. This sedentariness has the potential to become the beginning of a cycle wherein one's sedentary lifestyle precipitates further flexibility losses. The result is that the person becomes even more inflexible and responds by adopting a lifestyle even more sedentary than before.

Corbin and Lindsey (1994) indicated that flexibility in any given muscle group will vary depending on environmental conditions and the individual's psychological state. Variables affecting flexibility include motivation to put forth maximum effort, degree of relaxation, warm-up, muscle soreness, and environmental temperature. Particularly when assessing flexibility, the above conditions should be kept as stable as possible. Controlling such variables helps facilitate valid judgments when score comparisons are an issue.

Individuals with disabilities, perhaps because of inopportunity or lowered expectations of themselves and from others, may not be as flexible as the general population. Flexibility, too, is a function of muscle fitness. Typically, fit muscles, provided they have been exercised through normal ranges of motion, are flexible muscles. To the degree that one is not fit, inflexibility may be, in part, fitness related; that is, there are interactions among fitness components such as flexibility, skinfold, sit-up score, PWC 170, and grip strength to total fitness that are independent of age and gender (Fenster et al., 1990).

A number of disabilities often mitigate against flexibility. For example, spastic cerebral palsy is characterized by hypertonicity and contractures in affected muscle groups. How flexible the person with spastic cerebral palsy is at any given time may be determined, to varying degrees, by ambient temperature, level of arousal, and medication. An individual with spastic cerebral palsy who is in a warm room, calm, and taking muscle relaxers is likely to demonstrate more flexibility than if he or she were cold, excited, and not taking (or had neglected to take) prescribed muscle relaxing medication. Individuals with Duchenne muscular dystrophy often will experience decrements in flexibility owing to the dystrophic muscles' diseased state. Children with juvenile rheumatoid arthritis typically will be inflexible due to joint pain which mitigates against movement. This pain, to the degree it discourages movement, inevitably results in some range of motion loss.

Flexibility is highly specific. One cannot make generalizations about overall flexibility by measuring range of motion only at one site. In fact, the only valid way to determine range of motion in any joint is to specifically measure range of motion at that specific joint.

It is important to note that many flexibility measures, even some venerable ones, may be questionable in terms of validity. Take, for example, sit-and-reach as a flexibility measure. Given this case, at least three factors could influence the individual's flexibility score, and often it is difficult to determine precisely the degree to which each factor has contributed. Factors include back flexibility, hamstring flexibility, and arm length to leg length ratio. Further, the slightest flexion at the knee joint will render a sit-and-reach score invalid, because hamstrings, the major muscle group being stretched, cross the knee joint.

Flexibility scores may be reported as linear measures or rotary measures. Although each measure is efficient, linear measures probably have greater applicability in practical settings. Typically, linear measures require little more than some form of ruler or sit-and-reach box, in which flexibility of a particular muscle group (hamstrings) or range of motion (shoulder) is noted. Recently, Hoeger et al. (1990) recommended a modified sit-and-reach that incorporates a finger-to-box distance to control limb-length biases (see Figures 7.4 and 7.5). This test may be more

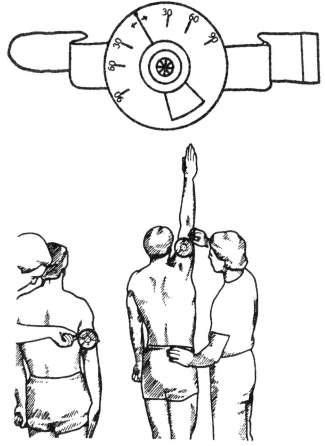

FIGURE 7.4 Flexometer

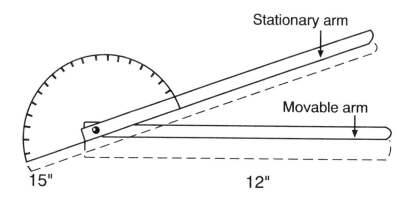

Stationary arm

Movable arm

15"

12"

FIGURE 7.5 Goniometer

appropriate for individuals with disabilities not only to eliminate limb length bias but to circumvent problems with excessive tightness or weakness associated with certain disabilities. Further, by utilizing specific tests of muscle groups such as the length of hamstring muscles (see Figure 7.6), the teacher/clinician can document the length of the hamstrings by ensuring that the back is flat, with one leg on the floor while raising the opposite leg (Kendall, McCreary, and Provance, 1993).

Rotary measures usually require devices or instruments more typically seen in laboratory settings (e.g., flexometers, goniometers). In addition, flexion and extension of specific movements (see Figure 7.7) can be used to document movement through an arc of 0–180 degrees. Specific flexibility can be determined through range of motion in the extremities, rotation of the limbs, or movements in planes around the horizontal, vertical, or coronal axis (Norkin and White, 1988).

Cardiorespiratory Endurance

Many people equate "being in good shape" with the ability to effectively meet challenges requiring cardiorespiratory endurance. Such challenges include, but are not limited to, bicycle riding, rowing or paddling, power walking, jogging, swimming, cross country skiing, and in-line skating. The ability to engage in these types of activities and have the experience be enjoyable typically is equated with "being fit."

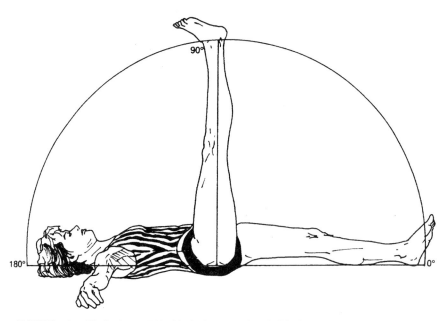

FIGURE 7.6 Hip flexion to 90° with the knee straight is ideal

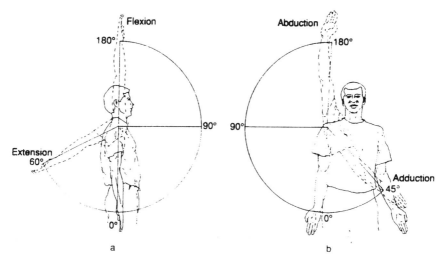

FIGURE 7.7 (a) Normal shoulder flexion-extension (b) Normal shoulder adduction-abduction

From Baumgartner, Ted A., and Andrew S. Jackson, *Measurement for Evaluation in Physical Education and Exercise Science*, 5th ed. Copyright © 1995 by Brown and Benchmark, Dubuque, IA. All rights reserved. Reprinted by permission.

Cardiorespiratory endurance arguably is fitness' most important component, particularly when potential for promoting health is the primary criterion by which fitness components are judged. Good cardiorespiratory fitness is considered important, given its potential for reducing heart disease and obesity risks.

Historically, the standard for measuring cardiorespiratory endurance has been maximum oxygen uptake ($\dot{V}O_2$ max). $\dot{V}O_2$ max, to be measured precisely, however, requires expensive and sophisticated equipment that simply is not available in the vast majority of practical settings. In order for $\dot{V}O_2$ max to be evaluated in practical settings without elaborate laboratory equipment and procedures, researchers have constructed tests whose results correlate significantly with laboratory assessments of $\dot{V}O_2$ max. Given that a field test for cardiorespiratory endurance correlates with its laboratory test counterpart, the field test can be assumed to validly measure cardiorespiratory endurance. Typical cardiorespiratory endurance field tests call for the subject to run a prescribed distance (e.g.,1 or 1½ miles) for time or run a prescribed period of time (e.g., 9 or 12 minutes) for distance (AAH-PERD, 1980, 1988). Other measures rely on pulse recovery following some prescribed level of exertion (Skubik, 1964). Some tests rely on cadence (e.g., use of a metronome) for standardizing workload. It should be noted that items requiring the individual to maintain cadence may be inappropriate if, for example, the person has a mental disability or attention deficit disorder.

A word of caution is in order regarding alleged measures of cardiorespiratory endurance using older test batteries. In the past, widely used fitness tests relied on either the 300- or 600-yard run as a measure of cardiorespiratory fitness (AAHPERD, 1976a; AAHPERD, 1976b; AAHPERD, 1976c). Distance runs of these lengths, however, have been found not to correlate significantly with their $\dot{V}O_2$ max laboratory test counterparts, and subsequently have been deemed invalid (Fernhall and Tymeson, 1988).

When pulse counting provides the basis for determining cardiorespiratory fitness, a number of considerations for the test administrator and/or test interpreter are in order. Pulse rate for any given level of exertion can be affected by factors including environmental temperature and the subject's level of arousal. Counting heart beats, particularly when pulse is rapid immediately following exercise, sometimes can be difficult. While post-exercise heart beats are being counted, pulse rate will be recovering towards normal. If post-exercise pulse is taken over too long a time period (i.e., one minute), the tester will record a pulse rate lower than that which was occurring at the moment exertion ceased. This is due to the pulse recovery phenomenon. To remedy this problem, most post-exercise pulse measures are of either six or ten seconds in duration. When pulse is taken for six seconds, the tester need only add a zero to the number of beats counted to determine beats per minute. When pulse is taken for ten seconds, the tester multiplies the number of beats counted by six. The major drawback to the six second method is that an inaccurate pulse count by only one heart beat results in a ten beat per minute error. Compact electronic pulse monitors are available, but may not be available in field-based settings.

Ideal places for taking pulse are at the radial artery (located immediately proximal to the wrist joint between finger flexor tendons and the radius) and the carotid artery (located at the side of the larynx midway between shoulder and jaw). Two fingers (do not use the thumb) with just enough pressure to palpate the pulse work best.

Certain field tests of cardiorespiratory fitness are more time consuming than others. By their very nature, most tests of cardiorespiratory endurance can be relatively time consuming. Often the number of persons needing to be tested and the degree to which those being tested can assist in their own scoring (e.g., counting heart beats) will determine the specific measure to be used. Generally, in practical settings, group tests like the 9-minute run for distance or 1 mile run for time are most time-effective, while Fernhall and Tymeson (1988) reported a .88 correlation between $\dot{V}O_2$ max and the 1.5 mile run in subjects with mental retardation.

Prior to engaging an individual in cardiorespiratory endurance testing, it is essential to determine that he or she is free from cardiorespiratory or joint disease. For example, individuals with Down syndrome, as a group, manifest certain heart defects or alantoaxial instability not seen in the population at large. Before engaging in cardiorespiratory endurance testing, the tester should consult with the appropriate medical personnel on answers to the following questions:

1. Does the individual have any exercise induced allergies, or respiratory or circulatory complications?
2. Has the individual ever experienced faintness, dizziness, shortness of breath, or chest pains during or after exercise?
3. Does the individual have any bone, joint, or spasm disorders that may be aggravated by testing?

In certain instances, the individual may use a wheelchair, hands, feet, or assistive device for testing. Any special circumstances germane to ambulation should be noted, and, in retest situations, the retest should be conducted under precisely the same conditions as was the original test. Wheelchairs, in particular, can have a significant effect on any timed test, whether the test alleges to measure cardiorespiratory endurance or speed. Wheelchair frame rigidity, weight, and state of repair are all critical factors. In addition, using a combination of arms and legs, as with a Schwinn Air-Dyne cycle ergometer, may elicit values higher than expected because of more muscle mass involved (Pitetti and Tan, 1990). Subsequently, variations in the level or extent of disability also may affect remaining or functional muscle mass. For this reason, comparing scores among wheelchair users often is of limited value. Further, if there has been a change in wheelchairs or a change in the chair's state of repair between tests, the two test results should not be compared.

One problem inherent in cardiorespiratory endurance testing is that the person being tested may be disinclined to endure the degree of discomfort necessary to produce a valid cardiorespiratory endurance score. In such instances, the tester must undertake to determine what motivates each individual, as often seen in run-walk tests (Lavay, Reid, and Cressler-Chaviz, 1990). In extreme instances, the tester may find him/herself running with and encouraging the individual(s) being tested. Obviously, given the latter scenario, group testing is preferred. Further, if the person administering the test is going to participate alongside the individual, that tester must be consistent with the applications of motivational devices and be physically able to complete the test.

Body Composition

Body composition, or body fatness, refers to the percentage of total body weight that is fat. All healthy persons possess some adipose (fat) tissue. Some fat is essential for energy storage, body temperature regulation, shock absorption, and as a carrier for certain body nutrients (Corbin and Lindsey, 1994). Essential fat is estimated to be approximately 8–12 percent for females and 3–5 percent for males (Hoeger and Hoeger, 1992; Wilmore et al., 1986).

A person 10–20 percent above their ideal weight is considered overweight. Twenty percent or more above ideal weight is considered obese. One major problem, however, with using weight only to determine over fatness or obesity is that weight alone may reveal little about body composition. Two people given the same height and weight may be vastly different in terms of percent body fat. For health assessment purposes, weight measures alone should be interpreted with caution, and fat measures typically are more useful than weight measures.

Even among some persons appearing to be at or near ideal body weight, weight alone as an indicator of body fatness can be deceiving. A person may be of expected weight for age and gender, but her or his weight may be comprised of too little muscle and too much fat.

Desirable fatness for good health alone ranges from 10–25 percent in adult males and 18–30 percent in adult females (Wilmore et al., 1986). An ideal body fat percentage for adult females is estimated to range between 15 and 20 percent. For adult males, the estimated *ideal* range is 10–15 percent (Eichstaedt and Kalakian, 1992). Ideal fatness promotes not only good health, but facilitates good physical and motor performance.

Some researchers believe that deriving *percent body fat* measures from children's skinfolds may not be valid, because formulas for estimating percent body fat have been derived primarily from measuring adults. Concern arises over the possibility that body density and fat content relationships may differ between adults and children. For this reason, a child's given number of skinfold millimeters may, instead, result in his or her being placed on a scale ranging from excellent to very poor. Alternately, a given number of skinfold millimeters may result in the child's being assigned to a given percentile.

The majority methods for estimating body fat are not applicable in practical settings. Among these are potassium-40 analysis, radiography, nuclear magnetic resonance, and underwater weighing. In practical settings, skinfold measures typically provide the most valid and reliable means for estimating body fat.

Taking skinfold measures in practical settings requires that the tester become skilled in using skinfold calipers. When taking skinfold measures, it is critical that each be taken at the exact site specified by the test. A skinfold measure is taken by grasping tissue to be measured with the thumb and forefinger and gently drawing it away from the subject's body. At a point adjacent to the thumb-forefinger grasp of the skinfold, the caliper is applied (see Figure 7.8). It is important to be sure that *only* skin and adipose tissue (not muscle) is being measured. To ensure that muscle is not included in the measure, the tester can ask the individual to flex muscles directly beneath the skinfold measurement site. If the tester does not feel muscles tensing between the thumb-forefinger grasp, he or she may be assured that muscle will not be included in the measure.

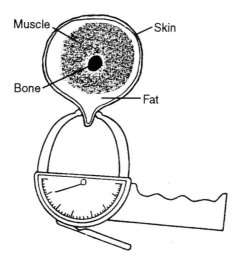

FIGURE 7.8   Measurement of skinfold fat

TABLE 7.2 Percentile Norms for Triceps Skinfold for Boys and Girls Ages 6–18

	Triceps Skinfold (mm)												
	Age												
Percentile	6	7	8	9	10	11	12	13	14	15	16	17	18
Boys[a]													
75	6	6	6	7	7	7	7	7	6	6	6	6	6
50	8	8	8	8	9	10	9	9	8	8	8	8	8
25	9	10	11	12	12	14	13	13	12	11	11	11	11
Girls[a]													
75	7	8	8	9	9	9	9	9	11	12	12	12	12
50	9	10	10	11	12	12	12	12	14	15	16	16	16
25	11	12	14	14	15	15	16	17	18	20	21	20	20

[a]Based on data from Johnston, F. E., D.V. Hammill, and S. Lemeshow. (1) *Skinfold Thickness of Children 6–11 Years* (Series II, No. 120, 1972), and (2) *Skinfold Thickness of Youth 12–17 Years* (Series II, No. 132, 1974). U.S. National Center for Health Statistics, U.S. Department of HEW, Washington, D.C.

Table 7.2 data (Johnston, Hammill, and Lemeshow, 1972) provide an example of interpreting body composition in terms of percentiles. Table 7.3 data (Pollock, Schmidt, and Jackson, 1980) provide an example of interpreting body composition in terms of percent body fat, and Table 7.4 data (Fahey, Insel, and Roth, 1994) provide an example of interpreting body composition on a scale ranging from excellent to very poor.

Katch and McArdle (1988, p.135) have developed the following formula that incorporates reduction of percent body fat into an activity program designed to facilitate achievement of desirable weight.

$$\text{Desirable body weight} = \frac{\text{Lean body weight}}{1.00 - \% \text{ fat desired}}$$

Given: A 200-pound male teenager has 25 percent body fat. The goal is to achieve a body fat of 18 percent. An example step-by-step computation to determine desirable body weight is as follows:

Step 1. Fat weight = 200 lb − .25 = 50 lb

Step 2. Lean body weight = 150 lb

Step 3. Desirable body weight $= \dfrac{150 \text{ lb}}{1.00 - .18} = \dfrac{150 \text{ lb}}{.82} = 182.9$ lb

Step 4. Desirable fat loss = Present weight − Desirable weight

= 200 lb − 182.9 lb

= 17.1 lb

Once the teenager loses approximately 17 pounds (assuming weight loss is, indeed, fat loss resulting from a combination of exercise and diet), he will have achieved his

TABLE 7.3 Percent Fat Estimate for Men: Sum of Chest, Abdomen, and Thigh Skinfolds

Sum of Skinfolds (mm)	Under 22	23–27	28–32	33–37	38–42	43–47	48–52	53–57	Over 57
8–10	1.3	1.8	2.3	2.9	3.4	3.9	4.5	5.0	5.5
11–13	2.2	2.8	3.3	3.9	4.4	4.9	5.5	6.0	6.5
14–16	3.2	3.8	4.3	4.8	5.4	5.9	6.4	7.0	7.5
17–19	4.2	4.7	5.3	5.8	6.3	6.9	7.4	8.0	8.5
20–22	5.1	5.7	6.2	6.8	7.3	7.9	8.4	8.9	9.5
23–25	6.1	6.6	7.2	7.7	8.3	8.8	9.4	9.9	10.5
26–28	7.0	7.6	8.1	8.7	9.2	9.8	10.3	10.9	11.4
29–31	8.0	8.5	9.1	9.6	10.2	10.7	11.3	11.8	12.4
32–34	8.9	9.4	10.0	10.5	11.1	11.6	12.2	12.8	13.3
35–37	9.8	10.4	10.9	11.5	12.0	12.6	13.1	13.7	14.3
38–40	10.7	11.3	11.8	12.4	12.9	13.5	14.1	14.6	15.2
41–43	11.6	12.2	12.7	13.3	13.8	14.4	15.0	15.5	16.1
44–46	12.5	13.1	13.6	14.2	14.7	15.3	15.9	16.4	17.0
47–49	13.4	13.9	14.5	15.1	15.6	16.2	16.8	17.3	17.9
50–52	14.3	14.8	15.4	15.9	16.5	17.1	17.6	18.2	18.8
53–55	15.1	15.7	16.2	16.8	17.4	17.9	18.5	19.1	19.7
56–58	16.0	16.5	17.1	17.7	18.2	18.8	19.4	20.0	20.5
59–61	16.9	17.4	17.9	18.5	19.1	19.7	20.2	20.8	21.4
62–64	17.6	18.2	18.8	19.4	19.9	20.5	21.1	21.7	22.2
65–67	18.5	19.0	19.6	20.2	20.8	21.3	21.9	22.5	23.1
68–70	19.3	19.9	20.4	21.0	21.6	22.2	22.7	23.3	23.9
71–73	20.1	20.7	21.2	21.8	22.4	23.0	23.6	24.1	24.7
74–76	20.9	21.5	22.0	22.6	23.2	23.8	24.4	25.0	25.5
77–79	21.7	22.2	22.8	23.4	24.0	24.6	25.2	25.8	26.3
80–82	22.4	23.0	23.6	24.2	24.8	25.4	25.9	26.5	27.1
83–85	23.2	23.8	24.4	25.0	25.5	26.1	26.7	27.3	27.9
86–88	24.0	24.5	25.1	25.7	26.3	26.9	27.5	28.1	28.7
89–91	24.7	25.3	25.9	26.5	27.1	27.6	28.2	28.8	29.4
92–94	25.4	26.0	26.6	27.2	27.8	28.4	29.0	29.6	30.2
95–97	26.1	26.7	27.3	27.9	28.5	29.1	29.7	30.3	30.9
98–100	26.9	27.4	28.0	28.6	29.2	29.8	30.4	31.0	31.6
101–103	27.5	28.1	28.7	29.3	29.9	30.5	31.1	31.7	32.3
104–106	28.2	28.8	29.4	30.0	30.6	31.2	31.8	32.4	33.0
107–109	28.9	29.5	30.1	30.7	31.3	31.9	32.5	33.1	33.7
110–112	29.6	30.2	30.8	31.4	32.0	32.6	33.2	33.8	34.4
113–115	30.2	30.8	31.4	32.0	32.6	33.2	33.8	34.5	35.1
116–118	30.9	31.5	32.1	32.7	33.3	33.9	34.5	35.1	35.7
119–121	31.5	32.1	32.7	33.3	33.9	34.5	35.1	35.7	36.4
122–124	32.1	32.7	33.3	33.9	34.5	35.1	35.8	36.4	37.0
125–127	32.7	33.3	33.9	34.5	35.1	35.8	36.4	37.0	37.6

TABLE 7.3—*Continued*   Percent Fat Estimate for Women: Sum of Triceps, Suprailium, and Thigh Skinfolds

				Age to Last Year					
Sum of Skinfolds (mm)	Under 22	23–27	28–32	33–37	38–42	43–47	48–52	53–57	Over 57
23–25	9.7	9.9	10.2	10.4	10.7	10.9	11.2	11.4	11.7
26–28	11.0	11.2	11.5	11.7	12.0	12.3	12.5	12.7	13.0
29–31	12.3	12.5	12.8	13.0	13.3	13.5	13.8	14.0	14.3
32–34	13.6	13.8	14.0	14.3	14.5	14.8	15.0	15.3	15.5
35–37	14.8	15.0	15.3	15.5	15.8	16.0	16.3	16.5	16.8
38–40	16.0	16.3	16.5	16.7	17.0	17.2	17.5	17.7	18.0
41–43	17.2	17.4	17.7	17.9	18.2	18.4	18.7	18.9	19.2
44–46	18.3	18.6	18.8	19.1	19.3	19.6	19.8	20.1	20.3
47–49	19.5	19.7	20.0	20.2	20.5	20.7	21.0	21.2	21.5
50–52	20.6	20.8	21.1	21.3	21.6	21.8	22.1	22.3	22.6
53–55	21.7	21.9	22.1	22.4	22.6	22.9	23.1	23.4	23.6
56–58	22.7	23.0	23.2	23.4	23.7	23.9	24.2	24.4	24.7
59–61	23.7	24.0	24.2	24.5	24.7	25.0	25.2	25.5	25.7
62–64	24.7	25.0	25.2	25.5	25.7	26.0	26.7	26.4	26.7
65–67	25.7	25.9	26.2	26.4	26.7	26.9	27.2	27.4	27.7
68–70	26.6	26.9	27.1	27.4	27.6	27.9	28.1	28.4	28.6
71–73	27.5	27.8	28.0	28.3	28.5	28.8	29.0	29.3	29.5
74–76	28.4	28.7	28.9	29.2	29.4	29.7	29.9	30.2	30.4
77–79	29.3	29.5	29.8	30.0	30.3	30.5	30.8	31.0	31.3
80–82	30.1	30.4	30.6	30.9	31.1	31.4	31.6	31.9	32.1
83–85	30.9	31.2	31.4	31.7	31.9	32.2	32.4	32.7	32.9
86–88	31.7	32.0	32.2	32.5	32.7	32.9	33.2	33.4	33.7
89–91	32.5	32.7	33.0	33.2	33.5	33.7	33.9	34.2	34.4
92–94	33.2	33.4	33.7	33.9	34.2	34.4	34.7	34.9	35.2
95–97	33.9	34.1	34.4	34.6	34.9	35.1	35.4	35.6	35.9
98–100	34.6	34.8	35.1	35.3	35.5	35.8	36.0	36.3	36.5
101–103	35.3	35.4	35.7	35.9	36.2	36.4	36.7	36.9	37.2
104–106	35.8	36.1	36.3	36.6	36.8	37.1	37.3	37.5	37.8
107–109	36.4	36.7	36.9	37.1	37.4	37.6	37.9	38.1	38.4
110–112	37.0	37.2	37.5	37.7	38.0	38.2	38.5	38.7	38.9
113–115	37.5	37.8	38.0	38.2	38.5	38.7	39.0	39.2	39.5
116–118	38.0	38.3	38.5	38.8	39.0	39.3	39.5	39.7	40.0
119–121	38.5	38.7	39.0	39.2	39.5	39.7	40.0	40.2	40.5
122–124	39.0	39.2	39.4	39.7	39.9	40.2	40.4	40.7	40.9
125–127	39.4	39.6	39.9	40.1	40.4	40.6	40.9	41.1	41.4
128–130	39.8	40.0	40.3	40.5	40.8	41.0	41.3	41.5	41.8

From Jackson, A.S., et al. "Practical Assessment of Body Composition." *The Physician and Sports Medicine,* Vol. 13, No. 5, May 1985.

TABLE 7.4 Body Fat Standards for Health and Performance

	Percent Body Fat	
Classification	Males	Females
Excessively lean	Under 5	Under 8
Lean (high performance)	5–9	8–17
Healthy	10–20	18–25
Moderately overfat	21–25	26–32
Obese	Over 25	Over 32

From *Fit and Well: Core Concepts and Labs in Physical Fitness and Wellness* by Fahey, Thomas D., Paul M. Insel, and Walton T. Roth, by permission of Mayfield Publishing Company. Copyright © 1994 by Mayfield Publishing Company.

TABLE 7.5 Body Composition Standards for Boys (Standards developed from data published by Lohman, 1987)

	Triceps + Calf		Triceps + Subscapular	
Standard	Σ Skinfolds	% Fat	Σ Skinfolds	% Fat
Very low	<5	<5.9	<9	<5.9
Low	5–9	6.0–9.9	9–11	6.0–9.9
Optimal range	10–24	10.0–19.9	12–21	10.0–19.9
Moderately high	25–30	20.0–24.5	22–29	20.0–24.5
High	31–39	24.6–31.0	30–39	24.6–31.0
Very high	≥40	≥31.0	≥40	≥31.0

This table is reprinted with permission from the **JOPERD** (Journal of Physical Education, Recreation and Dance), Nov–Dec, 1987, 99–100. **JOPERD** is a publication of the American Alliance for Health, Physical Education, Recreation, and Dance, 1900 Association Drive, Reston, VA 22091–1599.

desirable body weight. Body composition in children and youth are included in most physical fitness batteries and are commonly shown as percentile rank norms rather than specific scores. Since variations in water and bone minerals are apparent in children, specific equations have been developed for children (Lohman, 1982, 1986, 1987; Lohman et al., 1984). In this procedure, the triceps, subscapular, and medial calf are recommended for three consecutive scores while only the medium score is recorded. Scoring is provided for the sum of the triceps and subscapular or triceps and calf skinfolds (see Tables 7.5 and 7.6). In two investigations related to individuals with disabilities, Johnson, Bulbulian, Gruber, and Sundheim (1986) developed an equation for estimating body fat of 23 athletes with spinal injuries (paraplegia) while Kelly and Rimmer (1987) developed a predictive equation for adult men with mental retardation. In each case the aim was to provide estimates of body fat specific to each population that could generalize to overall physical fitness.

TABLE 7.6 Body Composition Standards for Girls (Standards developed from data published by Lohman, 1987)

Standard	Triceps + Calf		Triceps + Subscapular	
	Σ Skinfolds	% Fat	Σ Skinfolds	% Fat
Very low	<11	<11	<11	<11
Low	11–15	11.0–15.0	11–15	11.0–15.0
Optimal range	16–30	15.1–25.0	16–26	15.1–24.5
Moderately high	31–35	25.1–30.0	27–35	24.6–30.0
High	36–44	30.1–35.5	36–44	30.1–35.5
Very high	≥45	≥35.5	≥45	≥35.5

Power

Power or explosive strength is a combination of muscular strength and speed. It is demonstrated when muscles contract rapidly to overcome significant resistance. Power is called for in such skills as throwing, kicking, running (specifically, accelerating), jumping, hopping, and leaping.

Power in lower extremities often is measured by the vertical jump or long jump. Vertical jumping may provide a more valid power measure than long jumping among certain subjects, because the former requires less skill. The long jump clearly calls upon power, but, in addition, requires that the subject understand and be able to execute optimal lean and foot placement to ensure jumping the maximum possible distance.

While the vertical jump (in terms of skill) may be less difficult to execute than the long jump, it often cannot be scored with the same precision. Vertical jump scoring usually requires that the subject mark the wall immediately prior to jumping, then mark the wall again at the apex of the jump. Occasionally, height of the pre-jump chalk mark will be more valid than the apex mark. While the tester can ensure that the prejump chalk mark is indicative of the subject's highest reach, she or he has significantly less control over documenting where the chalk mark is made at the jump's apex. Conceivably, a mark alleging to denote the apex could be invalid, because it was made before or after the true apex had been reached. Further, the tester can do little beyond visual or verbal prompting to ensure that the subject is reaching as high as possible when the apex mark is made. One possible solution to this dilemma is to eliminate measurement dependent on reach. Alternately, the tester may mark the wall to indicate the subject's standing height. Subsequently, the tester would mark the wall at a point equivalent to the height of the person's head at the apex of the jump. This method is limited by the tester's ability to accurately judge where the apex mark should be placed and by potential for the tester to get in the subject's way. In other instances, an instrument that relies on a sonar beam

(Vertisonic-Lafayette Instruments) has proved reliable in documenting jumping ability in children and young adults.

Upper extremity power measures may be appropriate for all, and particularly appropriate among persons with significantly limited lower extremity function. Upper extremity power can be measured unilaterally by putting a relatively heavy object such as a shot-put or bilaterally by imparting velocity to a medicine ball in chest pass fashion. Depending on individual subject ability, a softball may replace a shot, and medicine ball weight may vary.

Should the shot-put item be administered, the subject should put the shot from a stationary position. This procedure reduces the likelihood that lower extremity movement, including skill needed to produce lower extremity movement, will contaminate the upper extremity power score.

The medicine ball chest pass is administered with the subject seated in a chair (the chair's legs are secured to the ground). Securing the chair ensures that it does not move during force application. Alternately, the chair's back can be placed against a wall to prevent the chair's moving. The subject, using both hands, holds the medicine ball to the chest. She or he then pushes and releases the ball as aggressively as possible. Upper extremity power is determined by measuring distance between the ball's release and landing points.

One dilemma encountered in using the above upper extremity power assessment items is that normative data either may be inadequate or unavailable. For example, medicine ball chest pass norms are available, but only on a limited sample size of college men and women (Johnson and Nelson, 1986). The norms dilemma ceases to be a dilemma provided the tester is interested primarily in individual improvement. Here, the individual would become her or his own norm. Also, where norms are unavailable but desired, the tester, given adequate subject numbers in her or his own setting, may develop local norms.

A Sampling of Fitness Tests and Test Batteries

This section is intended to introduce the reader to a representative sample of fitness tests. Some are relatively old, some are relatively new, and some have been more carefully constructed than others.

All tests should be subjected to the user's scholarly scrutiny. The tester must not assume that a test, simply because it has been published and currently is in use, is valid, reliable, and objective.

Tests presented here are not necessarily being recommended. Rather, they are offered with the writers' comments and constructive criticisms for the potential user's consideration. Whether *any* test is selected for use must be determined according to the test's technical adequacy, tester competence, information desired, and characteristics of the individual to be tested.

Hand-Held Dynamometry

Many therapists and educators have begun to use hand-held dynamometry as a reliable and objective means of determining functional strength. Hand-held dynamometry instrumentation is designed to quantify peak force output when manually testing various muscles (Bohannon, 1990). In contrast to applying a graded, subjective rating of 0 (no contraction) to 5 (full movement and resistance), which occurs when manually testing a particular muscle or muscle group (Kendall, McCreary, and Provance, 1993), hand-held dynamometry provides a quantifiable measure of muscle force, usually in kg of force or Newtons. This essentially eliminates the subjective and often unreliable values obtained with standard muscle testing.

Recently, there has been extensive research supporting the reliability and objectivity of hand-held dynamometry with able-bodied adults, able-bodied children, and individuals with neuromuscular disorders (Dawson et al., 1992; Horvat, McManis, and Seagraves, 1992; Stuberg and Metcalf, 1988). In addition, this research has been extended to investigate the reliability and objectivity of hand-held dynamometry in individuals with disabilities (Surburg, Suomi, and Poppy, 1992; Horvat, Croce, and Roswal, 1993).

Manual muscle testers such as the Nicholas Manual Muscle Tester (NMMT) (Lafayette Instrument Co., Model 01160) or MICROFET (Hoggan Health Industries) are hand-held devices for quantifying isometric muscle strength. The Nicholas unit can measure forces from between 0–199.9 kg, while the MICROFET shows force exerted in fractions of a pound. Each unit is placed between the test administrator's hand and the subject's limb. Muscle force is then determined by either a make or break test procedure. In a make test procedure, the dynamometer is held stationary by the examiner while the tested individual exerts a minimum effort against the device. This is in contrast with a break test procedure whereby the tester exerts a force against the tested person's limb segment until the tested person's effort is overcome and the limb segment gives or breaks. Bohannon (1988) recently investigated the reliability of make and break tests and concluded that because the reliability of make and break tests was similar (i.e., differing by less than 1.5 percent), one testing method could not be interpreted as being clearly superior to the other. He also found only slightly higher strength values when using the break test procedure (Bohannon, 1988).

To use the hand-held dynamometer with individuals with disabilities, one session should be used to familiarize subjects with the testing protocol, test positions, and instrumentation to minimize effects of practice efforts on test performance (Croce and Horvat, 1992). Subjects are placed in the appropriate testing positions and allowed practice trials with the instrument until they are able to perform the testing protocol on cue. Test positions for measuring strength are commonly based on those outlined by Kendall, McCreary, and Provance (1993) or manufacturers of manual muscle testing devices (Hoggan Health Industries; Lafayette Instruments).

According to Horvat, Croce, and Roswal (1993), to ensure consistency in testing, the tester should: (a) use consistent body joint and dynamometer positioning, (b) stabilize movements, (c) give consistent verbal feedback to subjects during data acquisition, (d) provide the opportunity for subjects to visualize tested body parts, and finally, (e) place the dynamometer perpendicular to the limb segment on which it is applied. The latter point is important to ensure that the measured force against the testing instrument is maximal. The procedure has been used with individuals having minimal experience with hand-held dynamometry (i.e., less than five hours of practical experience).

A final consideration for testing protocol involved numbers of test trials. Most investigators recommend from two to four trials (Bohannon, 1990). An advantage of multiple trials is that test variability can be observed and judgments made regarding sincerity of an individual's effort. This becomes even more important when testing individuals with disabilities in that variability in performance is often encountered with this population. Consequently, it is recommended that the mean of three trials of dominant and nondominant sides be used. The sum of several muscle groups or a composite of strength values is also recommended to aid in program planning and evaluation of subjects.

Hand Grip Dynamometer

The hand grip dynamometer is a device used to measure static strength. In this procedure, the subject grips the appropriate apparatus and squeezes as hard as possible to elicit maximal force. Similar scores can be obtained with a cable tensiometer or dynamometer to record arm lift, arm press, or back lift (Lafayette Instrument Company). Baumgartner and Jackson (1995) reported that static strength measures correlate highly with work productivity tasks and can be used to document strength values in specific muscle groups (see Table 7.7).

Bench Press, Curls, Lat Pull-Down

In order to measure strength or absolute endurance, a weight training machine such as the Universal Gym or Cybex can be used to determine the 1RM. In this manner the greatest amount of weight for the specific exercise can be documented. For absolute endurance, a specific weight can be selected, for example 80 and 35 pound barbells for males and females in the YMCA bench press and 40 pounds for men and 25 pounds for women in the YMCA curl test (Golding, Myers, and Sinning, 1989). Johnson and Lavay (1988), recommend the bench press for students 13 years

---

TABLE 7.7 Correlations between Isometric Strength* and Simulated Work Tasks

Work Task	Correlation
Shoveling rate	0.71
50-pound bag carry	0.63
70-pound block carry	0.87
One-arm push force	0.91
Pushing force	0.86
Pulling force	0.78
Lifting force	0.93
Valve-turning endurance	0.83

*Sum of grip, arm-lift, and back-lift isometric strength from data by Jackson.

From Baumgartner, Ted A., and Andrew S. Jackson, *Measurement for Evaluation in Physical Education and Exercise Science*, 5th ed. Copyright © 1995 by Brown and Benchmark, Dubuque, IA. All rights reserved. Reprinted by permission.

of age or older using a 35 pound barbell. The child repeats the action until fatigue or 50 repetitions for males and 30 repetitions for females have been completed. Substitutions for younger children and schools without bench press equipment can use the flexed arm hang or isometric push-up in which the body is held in the arms extended up position of the push-up until it cannot be held.

Scoring for 1RM tests commonly documents the maximal amount of weight lifted, while absolute endurance records the number of repetitions or time maintained in a position for the push-up. Other variations of absolute endurance can utilize a 50 percent RM to document the number of repetitions using bench press, curls, and lat pull-downs.

Lower Extremity Strength

Isometric, isokinetic, and weight training equipment can be used to measure strength in the lower extremities. The 1RM strength test can be used to evaluate the leg press or leg extension to document maximal values of weight lifted or moved. With individuals with disabilities, it may be advantageous to use manual muscle testing (Horvat, Croce, and Roswal, 1993) or utilize a 50 percent RM or 50 percent of 6RM to document the number of repetitions for the leg press, leg curl, or leg extension.

Upper Extremity Strength Measures

Several measures of upper body strength are usually included in fitness batteries. Procedures such as the flexed arm-hang and pull-up are the most widely used items. However, since these scores have a variety of problems, including zero scores and unaccounted differences in body weight, several modifications can be included. As mentioned earlier, Johnson and Lavay (1988) included the isometric push-up while other sources use a modified pull-up (Baumgartner, 1978; New York Modified Pull-Up, 1968; Vermont Modified Pull-Up, Ross and Pate, 1987). Performance in modified pull-ups is accomplished with an adjustable horizontal bar with the child's feet in contact with the floor. Hips and knees are extended while performing the pull-up (Woods et al., 1992). Children perform as many repetitions as possible to document strength and endurance of the arms and shoulder girdle (Baumgartner and Jackson, 1995).

Abdominal Muscle Strength/Endurance

The most common test used to measure the strength and endurance of the abdominal regions is the sit-up, usually performed for 60 seconds with the hands placed in a variety of positions. In the Health-Related Physical Fitness Test Battery (AAHPERD, 1980), the hands are placed on the chest while the knees are flexed to eliminate as much of the hip flexors as possible. Johnson and Lavay (1988) recommend terminating the test if the individual stops for four seconds, quits, or has completed 50 repetitions. They also recommend taking as long as needed to eliminate what was termed as the motor efficiency factor.

Flexibility

Lower Extremity Flexibility

The most common test for flexibility is the sit-and-reach that is included in most test batteries. Individuals sit with their heels flat against a 12-inch-high bench and reach as far forward as possible. Scoring is the farthest point reached on the fourth trial (AAHPERD, 1980).

Upper Extremity Flexibility

Hoeger et al. (1990) proposed an alternative sit-and-reach test termed the Modified Sit and Reach that includes a sliding measurement scale slid along the top of the sit-and-reach box until a zero point of the scale is even with the fingertips. This finger to box distance (FBD) establishes a zero point that accommodates the variations in limb length in children and may more accurately portray the lower limb flexibility in individuals with disabilities.

In addition Kendall, McCreary, and Provance (1993) assessed the length of the hamstring by placing the pelvis in a neutral position, anchoring the supporting leg, and using a staight-leg raising test. Normal hamstring length (70°–80°), excessive length (110°), and short hamstring length (50°) can be detected (as shown in Figure 7.6). This technique may be especially helpful in individuals with disabilities since range of motion or flexibility in joints may be linked to functional capabilities. For example, in paraplegia, tightness in some muscles enhances muscle function, while in quadriplegia tightness of lower trunk muscles aids in maintaining sitting postures by increasing trunk stability (O'Sullivan and Schmitz, 1988). In contrast, other groups require flexibility to complete many functional tasks such as transfers or dressing. Likewise, the excessive flexibility in Down syndrome may result in ligament instability that affects activities of daily living and muscle development or imbalances. Other functional measures of flexibility can utilize a goniometer to document range of motion in the joints or simply to document specific movements through a 180 ROM (as shown in Figure 7.7) during flexion and extension (Norkin and White, 1988).

In addition, rotary movement, as measured by the goniometer, can be used to measure head, arm, or leg flexibility in the frontal, horizontal, or sagittal planes (Norkin and White, 1988).

Further, Palmer and Epler (1990) have provided illustrations of functional muscle movements, such as hip flexion, in which the individual stands and places the foot of the test limb on an 8-inch step and returns it to the floor (see Figure 7.9). The examiner can document the movement through the specific range needed to climb stairs, or document muscle strength by the number of repetitions from 0 (nonfunctional) to 5 (functional).

Body Composition

Measurement of body composition is difficult in children and individuals with disabilities since most measures were developed in the adult population. Children's water and bone mineral content varies with developmental age as well as differences

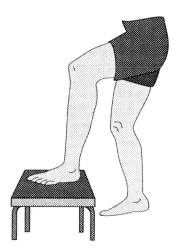

FIGURE 7.9 Hip flexion

in fat-free body density caused by disease (Lohman, 1989). Lohman (1989) reviewed several methods of estimating body composition in children, including the use of body mass index, anthropometry, body density, and bioelectric impedance. The following field-based measure of body mass index and skinfold measures are included.

Body Mass Index

Body Mass Index (BMI) is determined as follows:

$$\frac{\text{weight in kg}}{\text{height in meters}} 2 = \text{BMI}$$

Higher values for this index indicate higher body fatness. Lohman (1989) indicated that research on this measure found four correlations with skinfold measures and gave it a fair rating that should only be used when other measures are unavailable or impractical.

Skinfold Measures

The recent work of Lohman and colleagues provides a more useful measure of evaluating percent body fat in children. Body composition standards by Lohman (1987) include the sites of the triceps, subscapular and medial calf (see Tables 7.5 and 7.6). The sum of the triceps and medial calf are used in Physical Best (AAHPERD, 1988), FITNESSGRAM (Institute for Aerobic Research, 1992), and Fit Youth Today (American Health and Fitness Foundation, 1986).

Two variations that have been used for individuals with disabilities include an equation for adults with mental retardation (Kelly and Rimmer, 1987) using anthropometric data to estimate percent body fat. The Kelly and Rimmer equation is:

% fat = 13.545 + .48691649 (waist circumference) − .52662145 (forearm circumference) − .15504013 (height cm) + .07707995 g (weight kg).

Currently Rimmer has compiled a body composition data base on several hundred individuals with mental retardation using the skinfold measurements of the triceps, subscapular, and calf per the Slaughter et al. (1988) equation.

Another equation developed by Johnson et al. (1986) for athletes with spinal injuries (paraplegia) used circumference, diameter, and skinfold measures to estimate percent body fat in the following five models:

Model I (Anthropometric variables):
> percent body fat = 2.271 + 0.0754 (abdomen circumference in cm) − 0.305 (weight in kg) + 0.567 (chest skinfold in mm) − 1.017 (chest diameter in cm)

Model II (Diameter and length in cm):
> percent body fat = − 46.601 + 3.65 (Bi-Iliac) + 7.75 (elbow) − 1.145 (upper leg length) − 1.004 (lower leg length)

Model III (Circumferences in cm):
> percent body fat = − 33.535 + 0.831 (abdomen) − 0.587 (calf)

Model IV (Skinfolds in mm):
> percent body fat = 3.45 + 0.967 (chest) + 0.392 (calf)

Model V (Abdomen circumference only):
> percent body fat = − 31.804 + 0.617 (abdomen circumference)

Cardiovascular Endurance

One of the most difficult components of physical fitness to measure in children and individuals with disabilities is cardiovascular endurance. The amount of time, motivation, and ability to generate a maximal effort is difficult to sustain, causing the measures to vary with the population assessed. Some protocols will reduce the amount to be run/walked from 900 to 600 to 300 yards. It should be noted that these distances may not be sufficient to document cardiovascular fitness (Baumgartner and Horvat, 1991). Lavay, Reid, and Cressler-Chaviz (1990) provided an excellent review of measuring cardiovascular endurance of individuals with mental retardation. Fernhall and Tymeson (1988) also have investigated laboratory and field measures with individuals with mental retardation, while numerous authors have documented results with spinal cord injuries. In addition, Bar-Or (1983) has provided test data on individuals with cerebral palsy. Based on these investigations, the following field-based tests should be considered.

Run/Walk Test

Distance runs should be utilized to run for time or distance. Baumgartner and Jackson (1995) indicated that 1 mile and 9-minute runs are valid tests of cardiorespiratory function because they are related to maximum oxygen uptake and are included in Physical Best (AAHPERD, 1988). The 1 mile run is included on FITNESSGRAM. They also proposed using the 1.5 mile and 12-minute runs as alternatives, while the Fit Youth Today (FYT) battery uses a 20-minute steady state jog with the distance recommended as the criterion score (American Health and Fitness Foundation, 1986). Johnson and Lavay (1988) included an aerobic movement procedure that includes a run, jog, march, walk, propelling a wheelchair, exercise bicycle, scooter board, or walker. This procedure is included in Table 7.8 since it provides many variations for individuals with disabilities (Johnson and Lavay, 1988, p. 11–13).

Rockport Walking Test

The Rockport Walking Test (Kline et al., 1987) estimates $\dot{V}O_2$ max by walking for one mile as fast as possible and monitoring heart rates. Ross and Jackson (1990) developed a regression equation for estimating $\dot{V}O_2$ max based on weight (lbs), mile walk (time), exercise heart rate (beats per minute), and age. Pitetti, Rimmer, and Fernhall (1993) reported an equation for predicting cardiovascular fitness for the Rockport Walking Test as: peak $\dot{V}O_2 = 101.92 - 2.35$ (mile time) $- 0.42$ (weight) that was based on earlier investigations (Fernhall and Tymeson, 1988; Rintala et al., 1992).

Step Tests

The Canadian Standardized Fitness Test (CSFT) step test item, measuring cardiovascular endurance, has been modified by Montgomery et al., (1992) and Reid et al. (1985). The subject ascends and descends two 8-inch steps at a preestablished cadence, while heart rate is utilized to predict aerobic capacity according to the Jette (1976) formula. Depending on the heart rate elicited, additional 3-minute bouts of stepping are performed until the individual's target heart rate is achieved. It should be noted that Reid et al. (1985) reported that only 53 percent of subjects stopped the test because target heart rate had been achieved, and Montgomery et al. (1992) indicated that the CSFT overestimates peak $\dot{V}O_2$. Reid et al. (1985) reported lack of motivation tended to be a significant factor in subjects' failure to achieve respective target heart rates, a finding reported in many investigations of individuals with disabilities. Pitetti, Rimmer, and Fernhall (1993) have also indicated that muscular coordination and agility are variables that can affect step test performance.

Shuttle Run

Another test that has been used with individuals with mental retardation is the modified Leger and Lambert (1982) shuttle run. Montgomery et al. (1992) modified the first-stage speed (8.5 km/h) to 7 km/h before proceeding to the initial level of 8.5 km/h in the Leger and Lambert protocol. Pitetti, Rimmer, and Fernhall (1993) indicated that this modification underestimated peak $\dot{V}O_2$ values and measured anaerobic power rather than cardiovascular fitness, since participants must run at faster speeds. Pitetti et al. (1993) also indicated that muscular coordination, agility, pacing, and the type of floor surface can also affect the validity of this test.

TABLE 7.8 Aerobic Movement (indicator of cardiorespiratory endurance)

1. Administrative Procedures

In this particular test item the students may run, jog, march, walk with vigorous arm movement, propel themselves in a wheelchair, exercise bicycle, scooter board, use a walker, or move in any fashion to elevate the heart rate above the resting heart rate. The major objective for each student is to reach and maintain a heart rate between 140–180 beats per minute for 12 minutes after a six-minute warm-up. The tester monitors the student's heart rate every three minutes by taking a pulse rate check at the carotid artery for six seconds. If the pulse rate count is above 18 beats, the student is asked to slow down and is closely monitored for stress. *If a student's pulse rate is above 20 beats for two consecutive check points, the student is stopped and the test is terminated.* The student may change gait or means of locomotion throughout the test, but is encouraged to maintain the initial means of movement. It is recommended that no more than eight students be tested at one time on this test item. Keep in mind that it takes approximately six seconds to take a student's pulse rate at each check point. Allow all students six minutes of warm-up movement before starting the test item and use a record player or cassette for music with a fast tempo. The authors have also indicated that to eliminate motor efficiency bias, time and pulse rate are used rather than time and distance. Lavay (1993) also indicated that the test has been used with children as young as five years and is adaptable to a variety of disabilities.

Scoring: At each three-minute interval, scoring is determined as follows:

(1) First three-minute check (ninth minute; six-minute warm up + three-minute check)
Below 14—allow the student to continue to move, but give no credit. Student is encouraged to speed up movement.
Between 14–18—give credit for three minutes of aerobic movement.
Above 18—ask the student to slow down and monitor closely. Give credit for three minutes of aerobic movement.
(2) Second three-minute check
Below 14—allow the student to continue to move, but give no credit. Student is encouraged to speed up movement.
Between 14–18—give credit for three minutes of aerobic movement.
Above 18—ask the student to slow down and monitor closely. Give credit for three minutes of aerobic movement.
(3) Third three-minute check
Below 14—allow student to continue to move, but give no credit. Student is encouraged to speed up movement.
Between 14–18—give credit for three minutes of aerobic movement.
Above 18—ask the student to slow down and monitor closely. Give credit for three minutes of aerobic movement.
(4) Fourth three-minute check
Below 14—give no credit.
Between 14–18—give credit for three minutes of aerobic movement.
Sum the number of minutes the student has accomplished correctly.

---

*Note: A student is stopped when his or her pulse rate is above 20 beats for two consecutive checkpoints.
From Johnson, R., and B. Lavay, 1988—*Kansas Adapted/Special Physical Education Test Manual,* and Eichstaedt and Lavay (1992) Appendix D.

Power (Explosive Strength)

Power or muscular strength should be assessed in the upper and lower extremities. The Standing Long Jump is included in the AAHPERD (1976b) Youth Fitness Test, while vertical jump tests have been described by Beuman et al. (1988). The Sargent vertical jump test (Sargent, 1921) has the added advantage of adjusting the jump height to account for body weight. The Shot-Put (4–12 lbs) or Medicine Ball Put (6–9 lbs) Test can be used to record the distance thrown from a stationary position (McCloy and Young, 1954). Although not originally designed for individuals with disabilities, each of these tests seems adaptable to sitting in a wheelchair and throwing or pushing the medicine ball or shot-put.

Other tests that have been used to document explosive strength include the Wingate Peak Power Test (Bar-Or, 1983, 1993) and the Margaria/Kalamen leg power test (Margaria et al., 1966; Mathews, 1978). The Wingate test uses the arms or legs to pedal an ergometer for 30 seconds at a constant resistance. Power output is a function of the number of pedal revolutions in 30 seconds (Bar-Or, 1993). Bar-Or (1983) indicated this test was suitable for individuals with disabilities as well as children as young as 6 years of age.

The Margaria step-running test uses a series of steps (nine for adults and six for children). Power is based on the vertical distance, subjects body weight, and time to cover the designated distance (Bar-Or, 1983). This test is primarily a test of the lower extremities and has not been used with individuals with disabilities because it requires some skill to run the steps. Like the coordination problems evident in the vertical jump and standing long jump, this test should be applied to individuals with no physical limitations that would reflect on their performance.

Special Fitness Test for the Mildly Mentally Retarded

This test, originally published in 1968, provides national fitness norms from a sampling of more than 4,200 mildly mentally handicapped individuals aged 8–18 (AAHPERD, 1976a). This test was based on the original AAHPERD Youth Fitness Test first published in 1958.

A number of problems may arise with the use of this test. The softball throw item probably measures the specific skill of throwing being observed rather than any given component of motor fitness (i.e., coordination, upper extremity explosive strength). The agility run may correlate with mental age, thereby rendering its use questionable as a measure of motor proficiency. For years, straight leg sit-ups, because of their potential to injure the child's/client's lower back, have been abandoned as a measure of abdominal muscle function. Further, this specific sit-up item calls for the subject to alternately touch the right elbow to the left knee and vice versa. Some persons with mental disabilities may have difficulty comprehending or remembering the left-right sequence. The 300 yard run/walk is no longer considered an acceptable measure of cardiorespiratory endurance, because scores from this item do not correlate with known, valid measures of $\dot{V}O_2$ max. Finally, the test is currently out of print, norms are more than 20 years old, and may no longer be representative of current fitness levels among persons with mild mental disabilities.

Motor Fitness Test for the Moderately Mentally Retarded

This test was normed for use with persons aged 6–21 with moderate mental retardation, and is similar in content to the Special Fitness Test for the Mildly Mentally Retarded (AAHPERD, 1976a). This test's sit-up item was modified (i.e., bent knees) to reflect current thinking of the time. Here, the subject executes as many *bent knee* sit-ups as possible in 30 seconds (more recently, bent knee sit-ups have given way to curl-ups wherein the small of the back never leaves the surface). Unfortunately, the left elbow to right knee and vice versa aspect of the original sit-up item was retained. This test, like its predecessor, retained the 300 yard run/walk as its measure of cardiorespiratory endurance (AAHPERD, 1976c).

Norms are nearly 20 years old, and were developed from populations attending state schools for the retarded in Missouri. The age of the norms makes their use today of questionable value. Further, norms were developed in an institutional setting, and institutional settings typically have a depressing effect on test scores. In other words, persons who live in institutions generally achieve lower scores on a variety of measures than do peers who live outside institutional settings. Finally, while the test's sample size at first glance appears adequate (N = 1,097), actual sample sizes in some instances for a given gender and age are unacceptably small.

AAHPERD Youth Fitness Test

This test is a revision of the original which appeared in 1958. Norms for persons aged 9–17 were updated, and certain items either were eliminated or modified to reflect then current thinking. Three items measure health-related fitness, while three items measure motor (sport-related) fitness (AAHPERD, 1976b).

Although norms may be somewhat outdated, it is worthy to note that fitness scores have declined steadily in recent decades. The net result might be that if this test were re-normed today, any given item's 50th percentile might reflect poorer scores.

This test was not normed on populations of persons who have disabilities. For this reason alone, norms should be applied with extreme caution to anyone who has a disability. When this test's items are administered to persons from special populations, the tester should be certain that an item is measuring ability, not disability (e.g., the shuttle run should not be used to measure agility in one who has a significant visual impairment).

Bearing in mind the above caveat, tests of this sort can be used to facilitate placement decisions. Results can be used to help determine if the person's departure from typical population norms is sufficient to warrant placement in a special program.

AAHPERD Health-Related Fitness Test

Development of this test was based on the premise that fitness testing should focus on proficiencies directly associated with attaining and maintaining good health (AAHPERD, 1980). Proponents believe that fitness tests that include motor proficiency items measure little more than athletic ability. Their position is that while athletic ability is fine for some, it may be irrelevant for others. Further, they assert that having athletic ability and being in good health are not necessarily the same.

The Health-Related Fitness Test was normed on persons aged 5–17. Persons with disabilities were not represented in the development of this test's norms, therefore caution is in order when applying said norms to such persons. However, as with other tests normed on typically developing populations, this test's norms can be used with caution to help determine if the person with special needs might benefit from special programming.

AAHPERD Physical Best

AAHPERD recommends that this test replace *all* previous tests endorsed by AAHPERD (AAHPERD, 1988). This test, similar in intent to the AAHPERD Health-Related Fitness Test (1980), focuses primarily on health-related fitness. However, appendices within the manual also provide instructions and norms for measuring selected motor fitness components. Physical Best Test health-related fitness items are appropriate for persons aged 5–18. Motor fitness items appearing in the appendices are appropriate for persons 9–17+.

Performance standards are provided for each health-related fitness test item by age and gender. For example, in the 1 mile run/walk for 6-year-old girls, the standard is 13 minutes. The person tested can be deemed either to have met or not to have met a single performance standard for gender and age. The test does not provide norms that permit the tester to determine, for example, that a person's time in the mile run/walk placed him or her in the percentile. Percentile norms, however, are available for motor fitness test items appearing in the manual's appendix.

Where percentile norms are not available, Physical Best Test items are of somewhat limited value as tools for determining need for a child's/client's placement outside the mainstream. Typically, qualification for special programs requires performance below some specified level on a norm-referenced test. For example, if the percentile is determined to be a program's entry criterion, a person scoring below the percentile would qualify for entry. Since Physical Best Test (i.e., health-related items) does not provide such percentile scores, its use as a placement tool in some instances might be limited. Given this circumstance, the tester needing an instrument for placement purposes, with caution, may wish to consider one of the earlier published AAHPERD tests.

Physical Best/FITNESSGRAM

As this text is going into production, The American Alliance for Health, Physical Education, Recreation, and Dance (AAHPERD) and The Cooper Aerobics Institute are joining forces to provide for the physical education assessment and programming needs of persons who have disabilities. The forthcoming AAHPERD manual, *Physical Best and Individuals with Disabilities*, slated to be published in 1995, utilizes The Prudential FITNESSGRAM (The Cooper Aerobics Institute, 1992) Health-Related Fitness Test in partnership with Physical Best (Seaman, 1994). The manual will offer guidelines for modifying FITNESSGRAM test items or selecting alternate items, as needed, to meet assessment needs of individuals with disabilities. The manual also will offer curricula specific to meeting health-related fitness needs of persons with disabilities whose fitness needs may not be met in mainstream settings, as well as safety and measurement guidelines.

Alternate items for measuring aerobic capacity include submaximal assessments for some persons with respiratory and heart-related disabilities. Swimming, hand cycling, propelling a wheelchair, and walking are recommended as alternate items for persons with limited ambulation.

Suggested alternate body composition measures take into consideration the possibility that certain disabilities may preclude taking skinfolds according to individual need, and the person will become his or her own norm.

Suggested alternate ways of testing muscular strength, muscular endurance, and flexibility include any item with construct validity of which the individual is likely to be capable. Specific recommendations for persons with motor involvement call for elimination of timing factors on test items that otherwise would be timed.

Since FITNESSGRAM items are to be incorporated into the assessment facet of the forthcoming Physical Best/FITNESSGRAM program and are not norm-referenced, the assessment part of this package may not be useful for placement purposes. Generally, criteria for placement in a modified program will require a specific score (e.g., two standard deviations below the mean) on a norm-referenced test. Information preceding publication of the forthcoming manual (Seaman 1994) and The Prudential FITNESSGRAM (The Cooper Aerobics Institute, 1992) acknowledges this limitation. Their recommendation is that test scores for persons with disabilities, as appropriate, may be used for comparison purposes wherein the person becomes his or her own norm on key cutoff points, such as the 50th and 75th percentile, to make decisions concerning placement.

Physical Fitness Testing of the Disabled

This test offers norms for persons aged 10–17 who have auditory, visual, or orthopedic disabilities (e.g., spina bifida, traumatic paraplegia, cerebral palsy, amputations, congenital anomalies). Test items were drawn from the AAHPERD Youth Fitness Test and AAHPERD Health-Related Fitness Test. Norms are not applicable to persons who have either multiple or progressive disabilities. For comparison purposes, norms also are offered for persons who do not have disabilities (Winnick and Short, 1985).

Though normative samples were national in scope, sample sizes by age, gender, and disability often are quite small. The inherent risk in comparing one's children/clients to this test's norms is that scores from small samples may not be reflective of populations they allege to represent.

Kansas Adapted/Special Physical Education Test

One of the more recent tests for non-categorical assessment of individuals with disabilities who qualify for Adapted Physical Education is the Kansas Adapted/Special Physical Education Test (Johnson and Lavay, 1988). Test items include sit-ups, sit-and-reach, isometric push-ups, bench press, and aerobic movement. Test items were field tested on 200 children who qualified for adapted physical education in Kansas. Lavay (1993) has also reported that the items have been used numerous times in clinical and school-based settings with children as young as 5 years of age.

Because these test items are so adaptable to a variety of populations it is a test that should be considered. Group means on test items are available in other sources (Eichstaedt and Lavay, 1992). This test would also provide a fertile avenue for research and may be very applicable to school-based settings for documenting performance and developing program plans.

References

American Alliance for Health, Physical Education, Recreation, and Dance. *Special Fitness Test for the Mildly Mentally Retarded.* Washington, D.C.: The Alliance, 1976a.

American Alliance for Health, Physical Education, Recreation, and Dance. *Youth Fitness Test.* Washington, D.C.: The Alliance, 1976b.

American Alliance for Health, Physical Education, Recreation, and Dance. *Motor Fitness for the Moderately Mentally Retarded.* Washington, D.C.: The Alliance, 1976c.

American Alliance for Health, Physical Education, Recreation, and Dance. *Health-Related Fitness Test.* Washington D.C.: The Alliance, 1980.

American Alliance for Health, Physical Education, Recreation, and Dance. *Physical Best.* Reston, VA: AAHPERD, 1988.

American Alliance for Health, Physical Education, Recreation, and Dance. *Physical Best and Individuals with Disabilities.* Reston, VA: AAHPERD, 1995.

American College of Sports Medicine. *Guidelines for Exercise Testing and Prescription,* 3rd ed. Philadelphia: Lea and Febiger, 1980.

American Health and Fitness Foundation. *FYT Program Manual.* Austin, TX: American Health and Fitness Foundation, 1986.

Bar-Or, O. "Noncardiopulmonary Pediatric Exercise Tests." In T. W. Rowland, Ed. *Pediatric Laboratory Exercise Testing: Clinical Guidelines.* Champaign, IL: Human Kinetics Publishers, 1993.

Bar-Or, O. *Pediatric Sport Medicine for the Practitioner.* New York: Springer Verlag, 1983.

Baumgartner, T. A. "Modified Pull-up Test." *Research Quarterly, 49,* 1978, 80–84.

Baumgartner, T. A., and M. Horvat. "Reliability of Field-Based Cardiovascular Fitness Running." *Adapted Physical Activity Quarterly 18*(2), 1991, 107–114.

Baumgartner, T. A., and A. S. Jackson. *Measurement for Evaluation in Physical Education and Exercise Science,* 5th ed. Dubuque, IA: Brown and Benchmark, 1995.

Berger, R. D. "Relationship Between Dynamic Strength and Dynamic Endurance." *Research Quarterly, 4,* 1970, 115–116.

Beuman, G. P., and R. Malina et al. *Adolescent Growth and Motor Performance: A Longitudinal Study of Belgian Boys.* Champaign, IL: Human Kinetics Publishers, 1988.

Bohannon, R. W. "Make and Break Tests of Elbow Flexor Muscle Strength." *Physical Therapy, 68,* 1988, 193–194.

Bohannon, R. W. *Muscle Strength Testing: Instrumented and Non-instrumented Systems.* New York: Churchill Livingston. 1990, 69–95.

Clarke, H., and D. H. Clarke. *Application of Measurement to Physical Education.* Englewood Cliffs, NJ: Prentice-Hall, 1987.

Cooper Aerobics Institute. *FITNESSGRAM.* Dallas, TX: Institute for Aerobic Research, 1992.

Corbin, C. B., and R. Lindsey. *Concepts of Physical Education,* 8th ed. Dubuque, IA: Wm. C. Brown, 1994.

Croce, R., and M. Horvat. "Effects of Reinforcement Based Exercise on Fitness and Work Productivity in Adults with Mental Retardation." *Adapted Physical Activity Quarterly, 9,* 1992, 148–178.

Dawson, C., R. Croce, T. Quinn, and N. Vroman. "Reliability of the Nicholas Manual Muscle Tester on Upper Body Strength in Children ages 8–10." *Pediatric Exercise Science, 4,* 1992, 340–50.

Eichstaedt, C. B., and L. H. Kalakian. *Developmental/Adapted Physical Education: Making Ability Count,* 3rd ed. New York: Macmillan, 1992.

Eichstaedt, C. B., and B. Lavay. *Physical Education for Individuals with Mental Retardation.* Champaign, IL: Human Kinetics Publishers, 1992.

Fahey, T. D., P. M. Insel, and W. T. Roth. *Fit and Well: Core Concepts and Labs in Physical Fitness and Wellness.* Mountain View, CA: Mayfield Publishing Company, 1994.

Fenster, J., C. Ebbeling, L. Webber, P. Freedson, A. Ward, and J. Rippe. "The Effects of Age or Gender on the Interaction Among Field Fitness Measures in Children Ages 6–13 Years." *Pediatric Exercise Science (Abstract), 2,* 1990, 178–179.

Fernhall, B., and G. T. Tymeson. "Validation of Cardiovascular Fitness Tests for Adults with Mental Retardation." *Adapted Physical Activity Quarterly, 5,* 1988, 49–59.

Golding, L. A., C. R. Myers, and W. E. Sinning, eds. *Y's Way to Physical Fitness.* Champaign, IL. Human Kinetics Publishers, Inc., 1989.

Hoeger, W. K., and S. A. Hoeger. *Lifetime Physical Fitness and Wellness,* 3rd ed. Englewood, CA: Morton Publishing Co., 1992.

Hoeger, W. K., D. R. Hopkins, S. Button, and T. A. Palmer. "Comparing the Sit and Reach with the Modified Sit and Reach in Measuring Flexibility in Adolescents." *Pediatric Exercise Science, 2,* 1990, 156–162.

Horvat, M., R. Croce, and G. Roswal. "Magnitude and Reliability of Measurement of Muscle Strength Across Trials in Individuals with Mental Retardation." *Perceptual Motor Skills, 77,* 1993, 643–649.

Horvat, M., B. G. McManis, and F. E. Seagraves. "Reliability and Objectivity of the Nicholas Manual Muscle Tester with Children." *Isokinetics and Exercise Science, 2,* 1992, 1–8.

Jackson, A. S., et al. "Practical Assessment of Body Composition." *The Physician and Sports Medicine,* Vol. 13, No. 5, May 1985.

Jette, M., Campbell, J. Mongeon, and R. Routhier. "The Canadian Home Fitness Test as Predictor of Aerobic Capacity." *Canadian Medical Association Journal, 114,* 1976, 680–682.

Johnson, B. L., and J. K. Nelson. *Practical Measurements for Evaluation in Physical Education,* 4th ed. Minneapolis, MN: Burgess, 1986.

Johnson, B. L., J. K. Nelson, and M. J. Garcia. *Conditioning: Fitness and Performance for Everyone,* 3rd ed. Portland, TX: Brown and Littleman, 1982.

Johnson, R. E., R. Bulbulian, J. Gruber, and R. Sundheim. "Estimating Percent Body Fat of Paraplegic Athletes." *Palaestra, 3,* 1986, 29–33.

Johnson, R. E., and B. Lavay. *Kansas Adapted/Special Physical Education Test Manual.* Kansas State Department of Education, 1988.

Johnston, F. E., D. V. Hammill, and S. Lemeshow. *Skinfold Thickness of Children 6–11 Years* (Series II, No. 120, 1972), and *Skinfold Thickness of Youth 12–17 Years* (Series II, No. 132, 1974). U.S. National Center for Health Statistics, U.S. Department of Health, Education, and Welfare, Washington, D.C.

Katch, F. I., and W. D. McArdle. *Nutrition, Weight Control, and Exercise,* 3rd ed. Philadelphia: Lea and Febiger, 1988.

Kelly, L., and J. Rimmer. "A Practical Method for Estimating Percent Body Fat of Adult Mentally Retarded Males." *Adapted Physical Activity Quarterly, 4,* 1987, 117–125.

Kendall, F. P., K. K. McCreary, and K. P. Provance. *Muscles: Testing and Function,* 4th ed. Baltimore: Williams and Wilkins, 1993.

Kline, G. M., J. P. Pocar, R. Hintermeister et al. "Estimation of $\dot{V}O_2$ Max from a One Mile Track Walk, Gender, Age, and Body Weight." *Medicine and Science in Sports and Exercise, 19,* 1987, 253–259.

Kraemer, W. J., and S. J. Fleck. *Strength Training for Young Athletes.* Champaign, IL: Human Kinetics Publishers, 1993.

Lavay, B. (personal communication). "The Use of the Aerobic Movement Test for Children with Disabilities." 1993.

Lavay, B., G. Reid, and M. Cressler-Chaviz. "Measuring the Cardiovascular Endurance of Persons with Mental Retardation: A Critical Review." *Ex Sport Science Rev, 18,* 1990, 263–290.

Leger, L., and J. A. Lambert. "A Maximal Multistage 20m Shuttle Run Test to Predict $\dot{V}O_2$ Max." *European Journal of Applied Physiology, 49,* 1982, 1–12.

Leighton, J. "An Instrument and Technique for the Measurement of Range of Joint Motion." *Archives of Physical Medicine, 36,* 1955, 57.

Lohman, T. G. "Application of Body Composition Techniques and Constants for Children and Youth." K. B. Pantolf, Ed. *Exercise and Sport Sciences Reviews, 14,* 1986, 325–357. New York: Macmillan.

Lohman, T. G. "Assessment of Body Composition in Children." *Pediatric Exercise Science, 1,* 1989, 19–30.

Lohman, T. G. "Measurement of Body Composition in Children." *JOPERD, 53,* 1982, 67–70.

Lohman, T. G. "The Use of Skinfold to Estimate Body Fatness on Children and Youth." *JOPERD, 58,* 1987, 98–102.

Lohman, T. G., M. H. Slaughter, R. J. Borleau, J. Bunt, and L. Lussier. "Bone Mineral Measurements and Their Relation to Body Density Relationship in Children, Youth and Adults." *Human Biology, 56,* 1984, 667–679.

Malina, R. M., and C. Bouchard. *Growth, Maturation and Physical Activity.* Champaign, IL: Human Kinetics Publishers, 1991.

Margaria, et al. "Measurement of Muscular Power (Anaerobic) in Men." *Journal of Applied Physiology, 21,* 1966, 1662–64.

Mathews, D. K. *Measurement in Physical Education,* 3rd ed. Philadelphia: Saunders, 1978.

McCloy, C. H., and N. D. Young. *Test and Measurements in Health and Physical Education.* New York: Appleton-Century-Crofts, 1954.

Montgomery, D. L., G. Reid, and L. P. Koziris. "Reliability and Validity of Three Fitness Tests for Adults with Mental Handicaps." *Canadian Journal of Sports Sciences, 17,* 1992, 309–315.

New York State Education Department. *New York State Fitness Test: For Boys and Girls Grades 4–12,* Albany, NY: 1968.

Nordgren, B., and L. Backstrom. "Correlations Between Muscular Strength and Industrial Work Performance in Mentally Retarded Persons." *Acta Paed Scan, 217,* 1972, 122–6.

Norkin, C. C., and D. J. White. *Measurement of Joint Motion: A Guide to Goniometry.* Philadelphia: F. A. Davis, 1988.

O'Sullivan, S. B., and T. J. Schmitz. *Physical Rehabilitation: Assessment and Treatment,* 2nd ed. Philadelphia: F. A. Davis, 1988.

Palmer, M. L., and M. Epler. *Clinical Assessment Procedures in Physical Therapy.* Philadelphia: J. B. Lippincott Co., 1990.

Pate, R. R., and R. J. Shepherd. *Perspectives in Exercise and Sports Medicine* (Vol. 2) C. V. Gisolfi and D. R. Lamb, Eds. Indianapolis, IN: Benchmark, 1989.

Pitetti, K., J. H. Rimmer, and B. Fernhall. "Physical Fitness and Adults with Mental Retardation: An Overview of Current Research and Future Directions." *Sports Medicine, 16,* 1993, 23–56.

Pitetti, K., and D. M. Tan. "Cardiorespiratory Responses of Mentally Retarded Adults to Air-Brake Ergometry and Treadmill Exercise." *Archives of Physical Medicine and Rehabilitation, 71,* 1990, 319–321.

Pollock, M. L., D. H. Schmidt, and A. S. Jackson. "Measurement of Cardiovascular Fitness and Body Composition in the Clinical Setting." *Comprehensive Therapy, 6,* 1980, 12.

Rarick, G. L., and D. A. Dobbins. "Basic Components in the Motor Performance of Children Six to Nine Years of Age." *Medicine and Science in Sports, 7,* 1975.

Reid, G., D. Montgomery, and C. Seidl. "Performance of Mentally Retarded Adults in the Canadian Standardized Tests of Fitness." *Canadian Journal of Public Health, 76,* 1985, 187–190.

Rintala, P., J. M. Dunn, J. A. McCubbin, and C. Quinn. "Validity of a Cardiovascular Fitness Test for Men with Mental Retardation." *Medicine and Science in Sports and Exercise, 24,* 1992, 941–945.

Ross, J. G., and R. R. Pate. "The National Children and Youth Fitness Study II: A Summary of Findings." *JOPERD, 58*(9), 1987, 51–56.

Ross, P. M., and A. S. Jackson. *Understanding Exercise: Concepts, Calculations, and Computers.* Camel, IN: Benchmark Press, 1990.

Sargent, D. A. "Physical Test of a Man." *American Physical Education Review, 26,* 1921, 188–194.

Seaman, J. A. "AAALF and the Alliance: Partners in Fitness Education." *American Association of Active Lifestyles and Fitness Newsletter,* Vol. 1, No. 1, Fall 1994.

Shepherd, R. J. *Fitness in Special Populations.* Champaign: Human Kinetics Publishers, 1990.

Skubik, V. "Cardiovascular Efficiency Test Scores for Junior and Senior High School Girls in the United States." *Research Quarterly, 35,* May 1964, 184–192.

Slaughter, M. H., T. G. Lohman, R. A. Boileau, C. A. Horswill, R. J. Stillman, M. D. Van Loan, and D. A. Bemben. "Skinfold Equations of Body Fatness in Children and Youth." *Human Biology, 60,* 1988, 709–723.

Stuberg, W. A., and W. K. Metcalf. "Reliability of Quantitative Muscle Testing in Healthy Children and in Children with Duchenne Muscular Dystrophy Using a Hand-Held Dynamometer." *Physical Therapy, 68,* 1988, 977–82.

Surburg, P., R. Suomi, and W. Poppy. "Validity and Reliability of a Hand-Held Dynamometer Applied to Adults with Mental Retardation." *Arch Phys Med Rehabilitation, 73,* 1992, 535–539.

Tomporowski, P.D., and A.M. Hayden. "Employment of Individuals with Developmental Disabilities." G. Reid, Ed. *Problems in Movement Control.* North-Holland: Elsevier Science Publishers, 1990, 133–158.

Wilmore, J. H. et al. "Body Composition: A Round Table." *Physician and Sports Medicine, 14,* 1986, 152.

Winnick, J. P., and F. X. Short. *Physical Fitness of the Disabled.* Champaign, IL: Human Kinetics, 1985.

Woods, J.A., R.R. Pate, and M.L. Burgess. "Correlates to Performance in Field Tests of Muscular Strength." *Pediatric Exercise Science, 4,* 1992, 302–11.

CHAPTER 8

Assessment of Posture and Gait

The development of appropriate posture and knowledge of structural deviations that affect standing are essential to understanding movement problems. Posture can be defined as the manner in which the body aligns itself against gravity. Posture is influenced by the skeletal system, ligaments, muscles, fatigue, and the self-concept of the individual. Correct posture is achieved when all segments of the body are properly aligned over a base of support with minimum stress applied to each joint. Body positions that compromise the body's base of support and increase stress on joints precipitate faulty posture (Magee, 1987).

Posture encompasses more than maintaining a static position, since movement requires the body to consistently assume and change positions. Muscles that have sufficient strength and joints that are flexible will accommodate changes in position and adapt readily to stresses in movement. Chronic disease and faulty posture result as the body alters its structure to accommodate stress (Magee, 1987).

A sitting position with the back against the seat, feet on the floor, and thighs and back supported by the seat permits individuals to sit in a relaxed position while the chair provides body support. Additionally, when arm rests are positioned at elbow height, the arms rest thereupon to support and relax the postural muscles. Faulty sitting posture results in improper body alignment, slumping of the back and shoulders, and concentrating the majority of weight on one side of the body. Non-ambulatory individuals are especially susceptible to postural sitting faults and resulting complications such as pressure sores, scoliosis, and respiratory dysfunctions. The individual's specific disability and lack of muscular development and stability may restrict appropriate physical development and, in turn, stress joints needed to maintain proper sitting posture.

Standing posture is characterized by an erect position with an elevated head and chest, posterior-tilted pelvis, abdomen and lower back slightly curved, slightly flexed knees, and feet parallel and spaced a comfortable distance apart to allow for an even weight distribution. Various body builds as well as sensory or orthopedic impairments may affect the standing posture if proper alignment or structural components are altered and inappropriate stress is placed on muscles and joints. Improper standing posture may include slumping the shoulders, tilts of the head, protruding abdomen, spinal deviations or curves, and improper foot placement.

Individual Differences in Posture

When analyzing proper posture, individual differences that are associated with age, body type, and exceptionality should be noted. Infants and children in the primary grades may exhibit a wide base of support, slightly bowed legs, and a slightly protruding abdomen. Curvature of the spine that is common at this developmental age does not constitute a postural defect. However, the same occurrence in adult ages would indicate a marked deficit that may require corrective measures.

Specific body types and builds are more apt to assume various postures. For example, individuals may possess a mesomorphic, endomorphic, or ectomorphic body type, or any combination of the three body types. The upper torso may be the predominant characteristic of one body type classification, while the lower extremities may characterize another specific body type. The mix of body type classifications may lead to improper posture development, such as a muscular chest and back coupled with a slender abdomen and lower limbs that may appear as a rounded upper back. Orthopedic disabilities such as spinal injuries or amputations may also contribute to faulty posture if the disability affects the amount of muscle mass or alters body mechanics.

Causes of Postural Deviations

There is no single cause of posture deficits. Postural deviations can be either functional or structural. A functional condition may be overcome through corrective exercises or kinesthetic-awareness training of proper positions. Without proper maintenance of postural muscles and use of corrective techniques, the deficiency may deteriorate, possibly become debilitating, and either interfere with physical performance capabilities or become a structural deviation. Some functional causes of faulty posture include: (a) lack of muscular development, (b) muscular imbalance, (c) muscle contracture, (d) pain, (e) obesity, (f) muscle spasms, (g) respiratory disorders, and (h) loss of sensory input or proprioception.

Structural deviations occur due to abnormalities and/or deformities of the skeletal system resulting from disease or injury. Common structural deviations may include leg length differences, spinal anomalies, scoliosis, kyphosis, and lordosis. Because of the severity of structural defects, most are treated by physicians with a combination of braces, casts, surgery, and prosthetic devices. The assessment of posture and subsequent instructional programming should be interrelated to avoid potential problems and minimize effects of faulty posture on physical functioning. Some individuals with specific disabilities may demonstrate additional complications in walking postures such as shifting weight or regaining balance among individuals with a prosthetic device, a lack of proper feedback among persons with sensory impairments, and fatigue among individuals who use a wheelchair for ambulation. Persons with disabilities, as a group, have a greater incidence of postural defects than the general population. For example, lack of sensory information may contribute to poor postures or head tilts since the availability of sensory feedback is not used to maintain or reinforce appropriate postures. An individual with an amputation, spinal injury, or neurological disorder may place undue pressure on his or her postural structure while sitting and, in turn, may need to accommodate for balance changes and reestablish the center of gravity that is altered by injury or disability. For example, sitting upright is essential for performing functional skills and relies on the trunk muscles for spinal stability, while the imposition of a deviation such as kyphosis compromises achieving the upright sitting position (Meidaner, 1990). Without adequate strength in the trunk muscles, spinal deviations, low back problems, and mechanical efficiency for movement may affect the individual's ability to maintain an upright sitting position.

Assessment of Posture

In most instances, standing posture is assessed by means of a plumb line or by common instruments such as the New York Posture Test (New York State Department of Education, 1958), the Portland State University Posture Screening Program (Althoff, Heyden, and Robertson, 1988), or the San Diego State University Posture Evaluation, which is included in Table and Figure 8.1. If abnormal posture affects the ability to move or requires adjustment or compensations for movement, specific information must be obtained that provides answers on what is affecting the movement or posture. Posture assessment should also provide information about functional skill development for activities of daily living and for performing work-related skills. Posture problems may result from structural, sensory, mechanical, or neurological dysfunctions. For example, in an acquired deficiency, upright and walking posture may be distorted because of the necessity for shifting body weight and losing and regaining balance with or without a prosthetic device. Structurally, the base of support and center of gravity is altered, necessitating compensations in movement and posture to maintain an appropriate gait. Likewise, in recent spinal injuries, loss of function and subsequent time needed for various muscles to assume potential functions of non-walking muscle groups contributes to difficulties in maintaining a sitting posture.

As indicated earlier, loss of sensory function contributes to postural tilts in individuals with sensory impairments. Likewise, in acquired injuries the loss of sensory function and what may be termed "motor memory" may not be available to assume a posture or perform a specific movement. In incomplete spinal injuries and hemiplegia, the loss of motor patterns and muscle weakness may result from sensory deficit (Bobath, 1990). The resultant loss of posture is directly related to the lack of sensory information available for foot placement, tripping, or dragging the feet. In other situations, individuals may not be able to localize or locate sensory information, such as touch or pressure from slight to complete agnosia. Since the feel of the movement or limb is distorted, the individual encounters difficulty using sensory information to move the limb. Kinesthetic information does not provide appropriate feedback, thereby causing the limb to feel awkward and to be moved inappropriately.

A. <u>STRENGTH</u>

    1. Abdominal. See *Physical Best* (AAHPERD, 1988). (Modified sit-ups)

    SCORING: Record the number of curl-ups performed in one minute.

B. <u>FLEXIBILITY</u>

    1. Chest and shoulders. Assume hook-lying position. Keeping low back pressed to the floor (assistant should check by placing hand between lumbar area and floor), extend arms overhead and press back of arms and hands to the floor. Elbows must remain locked at all times.

    SCORING: ***WNL** — total contact of hands and forearms with floor
                    **LOM — contact of hands only with floor or cannot make contact without arching low back

    2. Spine and hip extensor. See *Physical Best* (AAHPERD, 1988). (Sit-and-reach)

    SCORING: Record the number of centimeters reached by the fingertips.

    3. Right hip flexors. Assume supine lying position with both knees bent over the end of a table. Pull bent left knee tight into the chest, keeping the right leg bent over the end of the table (Thomas Test).

    4. Left hip flexors. Same as above but with positions of the legs reversed.

    SCORING: **WNL**—if thigh remains flat on the table
                     LOM—if thigh lifts upward—estimate angle between leg and the table

Note: If thigh rotates outward or inward, rotators are tight. Star and report on the back of posture sheet.

          *Within Normal Limits   ****Limitation of Motion**

C. <u>ORTHOPEDIC EVALUATION</u>

    1. Foot examination. Note pes planus (eversion), pes cavus (inversion), achilles flare, hallux valgus, overlapping toes, corns, calluses, hammer toes.

    SCORING: Record degree of fluctuation. If greater than $1/4$ inch, indicates pes planus.

    2. Scoliosis check. "Procedures for Spinal Screening."

    FIRST: Ask if there is a history of scoliosis in the family.

    SECOND: Look at the students' backs while they are standing. Ask yourself:

          1. Head centered?
          2. Are the shoulders the same level?
          3. Are the tips of the scapulae the same level?
          4. Are the arms the same distance from the body?
          5. Are the trunk contours the same? Lateral deviation of spinous processes?
          6. Are the hips level?

TABLE 8.1—*Continued*

7. Are the popliteal creases level?
8. Are both knees straight?

The above are pieces of a puzzle. A positive finding in any of the above may be a normal variant or may indicate Scoliosis. The next check is perhaps the most important.

THIRD: The student bends forward with hands together, head down as if diving into a pool. View the student from the back. Ask yourself:

1. Is one side of the thoracic or lumbar spine higher than the others?

FOURTH: The student bends forward as above, but you view the student from the front. Ask yourself:

1. Is one side of the thoracic or lumbar spine higher than the other?

FIFTH: Take a quick look at the side view of the student as a check for Kyphosis. Ask yourself:

1. Is the curve even or does it peak?

NOW you make the decision for referral. The primary reason for referring a student is a rib hump which is usually accompanied by asymmetry of some type in the back.

3. Anterior view. Use a plumb line drawn from a point equidistant from the medial malleoli and extending vertically, bisecting the body.

   a. Head twist (lateral flexion combined with rotation to the opposite side)—torticollis
   b. Shoulder level—right or left drop of acromion process
   c. Linea Alba—right or left shift
   d. Anterior spines (hip)—right or left drop
   e. Legs

1. Internal or external rotation at the hip
2. Tibial torsion—patella face inward when feet are together
3. Knock knees (genu valgum)
4. Lateral view. Use vertical lines and estimate degree of deviation based on the following fixed check points: beginning with a point 1 1/2 inches anterior to the lateral malleolus and proceeding upward to the center of the knee (behind patella), center of the hip (trochanter), center of the shoulder (acromion process), and through the earlobe (tragus).

   a. Body lean—forward or backward
   b. Head—forward or backward
   c. Shoulders—forward or backward
   d. Kyphosis (thoracic curve)—use yardstick to check for perpendicular alignment to the floor
   e. Lordosis (lumbar curve)—measure the distance in centimeters to a vertical line (use yardstick) drawn between the thoracic and sacral apices
   f. Ptosis—abdominal protuberance, abdominal should not extend beyond a line extending down from the sternum
   g. Back knees (genu recurvatum), relaxed knees (flexed)

TABLE 8.1—*Continued*

5. Posterior View

    a. Head tilt—right or left drop
    b. Winged scapula—right and/or left
    c. Thoracic—right or left shift
    d. Lumbar—right or left shift
    e. Posterior spines—right or left drop
    f. Bow legs (genu varum)
    g. Pronated or supinated ankles—draw a perpendicular line from the ASIS of the hip to the floor. The line should pass through the center of the knee and between the first and second metatarsals.
    j. Short leg—note evenness of popliteal creases

D. DYNAMIC POSTURE

1. Walking. Observe walking front, side, and back view. Feet should be pointing straight ahead. The weight of the body should be taken on the heel first, then transferred to the outer border of the foot, then to the ball and finally pushing off the great toe. The body weight shifts smoothly and rythmically. Arms swing freely and in alternation with the legs. Note any peculiarities such as pronating ankles, inward or outward rotation of the hip, improper weight transfer, scissoring of knees, excessive trunk movements, stiffness, etc.

From Lasko-McCarthy, P., and P.M. Aufsesser, San Diego State University Fitness Clinic for the Disabled, San Diego, CA 92182. Used with permission.

Muscle tone associated with posture will also affect posture maintenance. Normal movements are supported by accompanying changes in posture and adjustments to movement, such as walking or running. In contrast, abnormal tone does not utilize the automatic adjustments in posture and movements needed for the tasks of walking or running. This can be seen in individuals with cerebral palsy, where spastic movements produce varying distributions and degrees of strength that interfere with purposeful movements.

The spastic muscle may provide excessive resistance or excessive assistance to movement (Bobath, 1990). These complications make it essential to observe changes in tone and movement response and relate them to changes in posture. For example, leaning to one side normally is associated with the contraction of the head and neck muscles on the other side. If the normal adaptation to this change in position is disrupted (i.e., the postural reaction mechanism is absent) the result may be a fall.

Bobath (1990) recommends placing individuals in a variety of positions with passive movements (see Table 8.2). The movements of adduction, abduction, internal and external rotation, flexion and extension, and supination and pronation should be used. As the limbs are moved to various positions, effects on posture and movement should be noted. For the practitioner, this can be a helpful screening device to note changes in posture occurring during movement. In normal posture, adjustments are made in corresponding muscles to adapt posture to specific movements. In abnormal posture, the lack of adjustment is noted, while some resistance may be encountered in some body segments such as the elbow, shoulder, hip, knee,

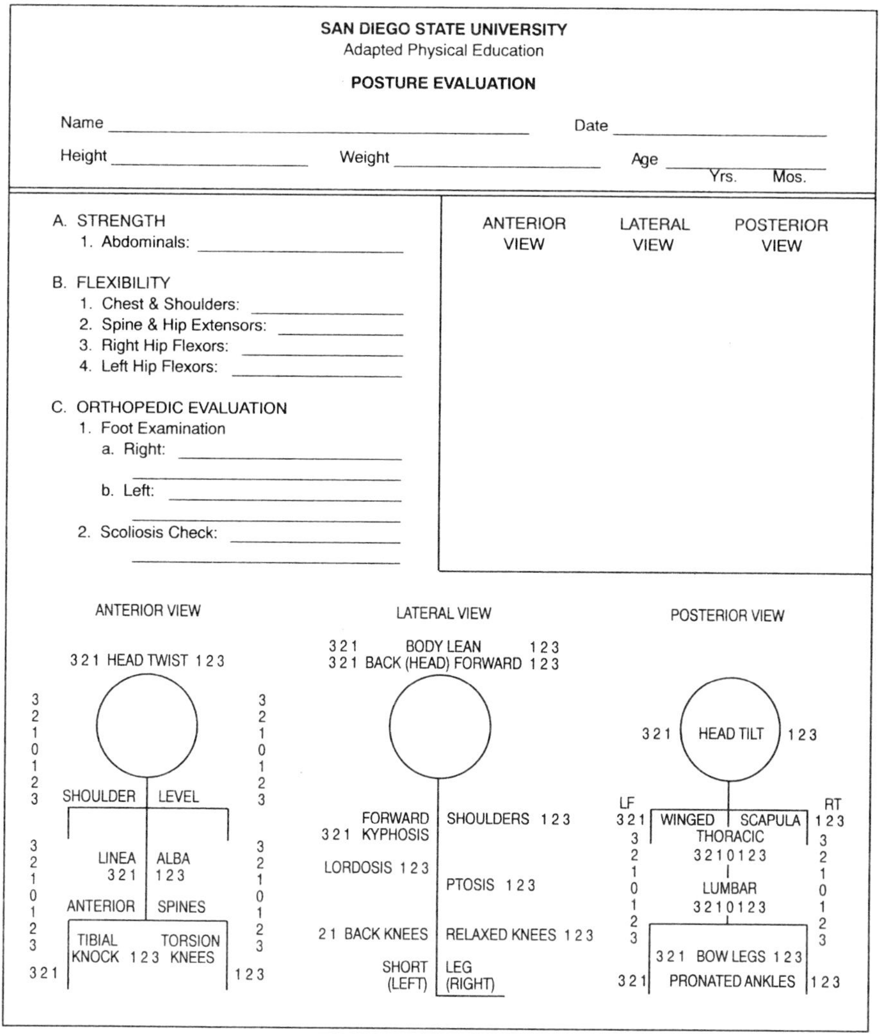

SAN DIEGO STATE UNIVERSITY
Adapted Physical Education

POSTURE EVALUATION

Name _____ Date _____

Height _____ Weight _____ Age _____
                                                    Yrs.   Mos.

A. STRENGTH
   1. Abdominals: _____

B. FLEXIBILITY
   1. Chest & Shoulders: _____
   2. Spine & Hip Extensors: _____
   3. Right Hip Flexors: _____
   4. Left Hip Flexors: _____

C. ORTHOPEDIC EVALUATION
   1. Foot Examination
      a. Right: _____

      b. Left: _____

   2. Scoliosis Check: _____

ANTERIOR VIEW	LATERAL VIEW	POSTERIOR VIEW

ANTERIOR VIEW

3 2 1 HEAD TWIST 1 2 3

3 2 1 0 1 2 3   3 2 1 0 1 2 3
SHOULDER | LEVEL

3 2 1 0 1 2 3
LINEA | ALBA
3 2 1 | 1 2 3
ANTERIOR | SPINES
TIBIAL | TORSION
KNOCK 1 2 3 KNEES
3 2 1 | 1 2 3

LATERAL VIEW

3 2 1 BODY LEAN 1 2 3
3 2 1 BACK (HEAD) FORWARD 1 2 3

FORWARD | SHOULDERS 1 2 3
3 2 1 KYPHOSIS

LORDOSIS 1 2 3
PTOSIS 1 2 3

2 1 BACK KNEES | RELAXED KNEES 1 2 3

SHORT | LEG
(LEFT) | (RIGHT)

POSTERIOR VIEW

3 2 1 HEAD TILT 1 2 3

LF 3 2 1 WINGED | SCAPULA 1 2 3 RT
3 | THORACIC | 3
2 | 3 2 1 0 1 2 3 | 2
1 | | 1
0 | LUMBAR | 0
1 | 3 2 1 0 1 2 3 | 1
2 | | 2
3 | | 3

3 2 1 BOW LEGS 1 2 3
3 2 1 PRONATED ANKLES 1 2 3

FIGURE 8.1 San Diego State University Adapted Physical Education—
Posture Evaluation

or ankle. Directional movement, especially in spasticity, may provide uncontrolled assistance as in a sudden pull or push. Moderate to slight spasticity may show assistance at the end of the movement, while in flaccid movements no active adjustments are indicated (Bobath, 1990). Since the muscles do not respond to postural changes, there are indications of postural reflex activity that results in the inability to perform active movements. For the teacher or recreational leader, this may indicate that the inability to perform a movement or task is specific to the lack of responses to postural changes.

In other cases, the sitting postures assumed by children with motor impairments may be directly related to the position assumed and trunk strength. For example,

TABLE 8.2 Test for Quality of Movement Patterns

Patterns to be Tested
Tests for Arm and Shoulder Girdle (to be tested separately in supine, sitting, and standing, as the result will be different in these positions).

Grade 1

	Supine		Sitting		Standing	
	Yes	No	Yes	No	Yes	No
a. Hold arm extended in elevation after having it placed there?						
With internal rotation?.						
With external rotation?						
b. Lower the extended arm from the position of elevation to the horizontal plane and back again to elevation?						
Forward-downward?.						
Sideways-downward?.						
With internal rotation?.						
With external rotation?.						
b. Lower the extended arm from the position of elevation to the horizontal plane and back again to elevation?.						
Forward-downward?.						
Sideways-downward?.						
With internal rotation?.						
With external rotation?.						
c. Move the extended abducted arm from the horizontal plane to the side of the body and back again to the horizontal plane?						
With internal rotation?.						
With external rotation?						
Grade 2						
a. Lift arm to touch the opposite shoulder?.						
With palm of hand?.						
With supination?.						

TABLE 8.2–*Continued*

	Supine		Sitting		Standing	
	Yes	No	Yes	No	Yes	No
b. Bend elbow with the arm in elevation to touch the top of the head?.						
With pronation?.						
With supination?						
c. Fold hands behind the head with both elbows in horizontal abduction?.						
With wrist flexed?						
With wrist extended?.						
Grade 3						
a. Supinate the forearm and wrist?.						
Without side-flexion of trunk on the affected side?.						
With flexed elbow and flexed fingers?.						
With extended elbow and extended fingers?. . .						
b. Pronate forearm without adduction of arm and shoulder?.						
c. Externally rotate extended arm?.						
(i) in horizontal abducton?.						
(ii) by the side of the body?.						
(iii) in elevation?.						
d. Bend and extend elbow in supination to touch the shoulder of the same side? Starting with:						
(i) arm by the side of the body?.						
(ii) horizontal abduction of the arm?.						

TABLE 8.2—*Continued*

Test for Pelvis, Leg, and Foot
Sitting Tests on Chair

	Yes?	No?

Grade 1

a. Adduct and abduct leg, foot on ground?. . . . .

b. Adduct and abduct affected leg, foot lifted off ground?. . . . .

Grade 2

a. Lift affected leg and place foot on sound knee? (without
   use of hand to lift leg?) . . . .

b. Draw affected foot back under chair, heel on the floor?. . . .

c. Stand up with sound foot in front of affected one? . . . .
   (without use of hand?)

Standing Tests

Grade 1

Stand with parallel feet, feet touching?. . . . .

Grade 2

a. Stand on affected leg, lifting sound one?. . . . .

b. Stand on affected leg, sound one lifted, and bend and
   extend standing leg? . . . .

c. Stand in step position, weight forward on affected leg,
   sound leg behind on the toes? . . . .

d. Stand in step position, sound leg forward with weight on it,
   affected leg behind and bend knee on affected leg without
   taking toes off ground?. . . . .

Grade 3

a. Stand in step position, weight forward on sound leg,
   affected leg behind and lift foot without bending hip
   of affected leg? . . . .

Foot in inversion?. . . . .

Foot in eversion?. . . . .

TABLE 8.2—*Continued*

	Yes?	No?
b. Stand on affected leg and transfer weight over it to make step with sound leg?		
Forward?		
Backward?		
c. Stand on sound leg and make step forward with affected leg without hitching pelvis up?		
d. Stand on sound leg and make step backward with affected leg without hitching pelvis up?		
e. Stand on affected leg and lift toes?		

Adapted from Bobath, B. "Test for Quality of Movement Patterns." *Adult Hemiplegia: Evaluation and Treatment,* 3rd ed. Butterworth-Heinemann, Ltd., London, 1990, 35–42.

Meidaner (1990) describes straight sitting as pelvis rotated forward, weight over the ischial tuberosities, back straight, and lumbar spine moved toward lordosis; anterior sitting as trunk straight, weight anterior to the ischial tuberosities; posterior sitting as spinal kyphosis and pelvis rotated back and posterior to the ischial tuberosities. Meidaner (1990), using the modified Schober Measurement of Spinal Extension (American Academy of Orthopedic Surgeons, 1975), compared sitting positions on the floor, bench, and Ther-A Chair. It was reported that sitting positions with anterior sitting postures increased trunk extension. This finding is noteworthy since increases in maintaining the postural position dramatically affect the level of functional ability. Since the trunk muscles are essential for postural control in a seated position, strengthening these muscles and maintaining an appropriate position will allow functional capabilities, such as pulmonary functions and position changes, to fulfill daily living needs.

Further, the advancement of activities of daily living and work productivity should be addressed to determine if postural difficulties are interfering with functional performance. For instance, if lack of sensory feedback interferes with a manual task necessary to complete a job or to learn grooming skills, adjustments or compensations in other sensory modalities should be implemented. For example, if kinesthetic feedback cannot be used to aid in combing an individual's hair, manual prompting or using vision are ways to cue the proper position. Likewise, variations of head control may interfere with computer skills and communication. If functioning is impeded by adjustments or lack of adjustments to the body, the assessment of posture and muscle tone should be implemented. Adequate assessments should be helpful in addressing posture-related movement problems commonly seen in individuals with disabilities. Included in Table 8.2 is the Test for Quality of Movement Patterns adapted from Bobath (1990). Although this assessment was developed for individuals with hemiplegia, the teacher or recreational leader can use responses to these movements to address postural deviations that affect movement potential. This information can then be used in conjunction with a standard static posture assessment such as the New York Posture Test, the Portland State University Screening Program, and the San Diego State Posture Evaluation to generate an accurate assessment of posture. Teachers or recreational leaders can then base their instructional programs on activities designed to alleviate these problems.

Gait Analysis

Developmentally, posture is the parameter that affects transition from standing to movements such as walking or running. It may be adequate to stand, but vary undesirably in walking or running if the individual does not have adequate maturity, balance, or strength to maintain an upright posture while walking or running. According to Clark and Whitall (1989), forces that are created in running may stress the postural system's ability to maintain an upright position. Since running uses the same pattern of intralimb coordination as creeping or walking, difficulty in maintaining postures during movements such as running are viewed as an upscale of force production that may pose difficulties for immature individuals and individuals with disabilities.

Because of poor development and postural instability, children with disabilities have difficulties in making transitions between basic locomotor patterns, being unable to deal with the increase in force production (Horvat, 1990). Thelen, Ulrich, and Jensen (1989) describe the transition from nonambulatory movements to walking by stressing the need for adequate balance and stability before the underlying coordinative patterns of walking become apparent. Difficulty in developing these components does not allow for the step cycle to be initiated or for adjustments to changes in the environment, such as variations in terrain. Unless the individual develops a combination of strength and stability, independent walking will not be achieved. Likewise, disorders that affect these underlying coordinative structures, such as cerebral palsy, change basic locomotor parameters. For example, the normal order of hip movements in walking is flexion, abduction, and external rotation. In spasticity, movements are flexion, adduction, and internal rotation (Sudgen and Keogh, 1990). Movement difficulties may result from some underlying factors that should be assessed to adequately portray the developmental needs of the individual. The observation that the child cannot run should be more thoroughly investigated to ascertain the specific components that may be interfering with or delaying development of the appropriate movement pattern or sequence.

In clinical settings, there are a variety of techniques used for gait analysis that evaluate muscle functions and correlate them with gait. Most comprehensive gait assessments are conducted with electromyographs for muscle function and force plates to record forces and torques on body segments (Vaughan, Davis, and O'Connor,

1992). Although this information is beneficial, most field-based assessments will rely on observational data and videotapes of gaits to detect abnormalities. These latter techniques should be sufficient to detect problem areas in strength and posture that affect ambulation and development patterns.

Assessment

The observation of functional gait patterns is used quite extensively in clinical settings. Observational assessments such as those used by Temple University (Bampton, 1979), Rancho Los Amigos Medical Center (Gronley and Perry, 1993), and the Gait Analysis Laboratory (Vaughan, Davis, and O'Connor, 1992) direct attention to a specific body segment at a point during a gait cycle. For example, the tester may observe heel striking at that point during a gait cycle to determine if normal or abnormal movements are occurring during walking.

Scoring may vary from the Temple University system of present, inconsistent, borderline, occurs throughout, absent, limited, and/or exaggerated for 48 gait deviations, to the Rancho Los Amigos system of assessing movements of body segments in the gait cycle: ankle, foot, knee, hip, pelvis, and trunk (Los Amigos Research and Education Institute, 1993). This evaluation also consists of 48 gait deviations such as hip hiking, varus or valgus, and/or toe dragging.

Vaughan et al. (1992) is the newest application to gait analysis with the computerized software package developed in conjunction with Human Kinetics Publishers. Although the framework is designed for biomechanical analysis, the framework of this program provides basic kinematics and muscle responses that can be used to functionally assess gait parameters. For the practitioner, observation of the movement pattern is the most useful and functional way to detect gait abnormalities. In order to conduct a gait analysis in a field-based instructional or recreational setting, it is recommended that the tester become familiar with the Normal Gait, Normal Gait Terminology, Normal Gait Cycle, and Abnormal Gait sections before applying the analysis to the Detecting Gait Abnormalities.

Because observational gait analysis is subjective and requires quick decisions, it is recommended that the individual's patterns be videotaped to provide a complete analysis of the entire body and sufficient time to document the individual's movement process. The taping procedure also aids in determining reliability within the observational assessment.

Normal Gait and Gait Terminology

In order to adequately assess deviations in gait patterns, an understanding of gait terminology (see Table 8.3) and the normal pattern should be recognized (Magee, 1987; Norkin, 1988). Developmentally, changes in gait patterns are achieved as early as 2 years for an advanced pattern. Pelvic rotation is usually evident at 13.8 months, knee flexion mid-support at 16.3 months, base of support at 17 months, and heel and forefoot strike at 18.5 months (Payne and Issacs, 1995). Obviously, growth parameters will increase the stride length and stepping rate, while normal walking should be well ingrained and functional at 7 years of age.

TABLE 8.3 Gait Terminology

Gait cycle	time interval or sequence of motions between two contracts of the same foot
Stride	one complete gait cycle
Step	beginning of sequence by one limb until beginning of sequence with the contralateral limb
Stance phase	foot is on the ground bearing weight allowing lower leg to support body and advancement of the body over the supporting limb—makes up 60 percent of gait cycle and consists of 5 subphases: 1. initial contact (heel strike) 2. load response (foot flat) 3. midstance (single-leg stance) 4. terminal stance (heel-off) 5. preswing (toe-off)
Swing phase	foot is moving forward and not bearing weight—allows toes to clear floor and adjust the leg as well as advancing the swing leg forward approximately 40 percent of gait cycle and consists of three subphases: 1. initial swing (acceleration) 2. midswing 3. terminal swing (deceleration)
Double stance	phase when parts of both feet are on the ground consisting of 25 percent of gait cycle
Single leg stance	phase when one leg is on the ground, occurring twice during gait cycle making up approximately 30 percent of gait cycle
Base width	distance between two feet x 5 to 10 cm varies with poor balance, loss of sensation and proprioception
Step length	distance between successive contract points in opposite feet x 35 to 41 cm varies with age, height, fatigue, pain, and disease
Stride length	linear distance between successive points of contact of the same foot, approximately 70 to 80 cm and is a gait cycle
Pelvic shift	side to side (lateral) of pelvis necessary to align weight over stance leg
Pelvic rotation	rotation of pelvis to lessen angle of femur with the floor to aid in regulating individual's speed of walking and decreasing center of gravity
Cadence	number of steps per minute from heel strike to toe-off, approximately 90–120 per minute

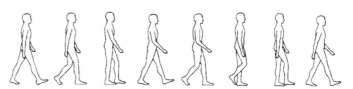

	Weight Acceptance		Single Limb Support		Swing Limb Advancement			
Reference Limb	**IC**	**LR**	**MSt**	**TSt**	**PSw**	**ISw**	**MSw**	**TSw**
Opposite Limb	PSw	PSw	ISw/MSw	TSw	IC/LR	MSt	MSt	TSt
TRUNK	Erect ———————————————————————————————————————→							
PELVIS	5° Fwd Rotation	5° Fwd Rotation	0°	5° Bkwd Rotation	5° Bkwd Rotation	5° Bkwd Rotation	0°	5° Fwd Rotation
HIP	25° Flex	25° Flex	0°	20° Apparent Hyperext	0°	15° Flex	25° Flex	25° Flex
KNEE	0°	15° Flex	0°	0°	40° Flex	60° Flex	25° Flex	0°
ANKLE	0°	10° Plantar Flex	5° Dorsiflex	10° Dorsiflex	20° Plantar Flex	10° Plantar Flex	0°	0°
TOES	0°	0°	0°	30° MTP Ext	60° MTP Ext	0°	0°	0°

FIGURE 8.2   Range of Motion Summary

From *Observational Gait Analysis,* Rancho Los Amigos Medical Center Research and Education Institute, 1993.

Normal Gait Cycle

In a normal gait cycle (see Figure 8.2), the swing and stance phases can be noted (Magee, 1987; Norkin, 1988; Soderberg, 1986). In the swing phase the initial swing is the first subphase. Flexion of the hip and knee allow for initial acceleration and stabilization of the trunk in single support. The ankle will plantarflex while the dorsiflexors aid the foot in clearing the supporting surface. At midswing the hip continues to flex and medially rotate while the knee flexes. The body is aligned in a single support phase with the pelvis and trunk. Maximum knee flexion is evident as the leg moves forward, ending the acceleration phase and beginning to decelerate. The terminal swing is the last phase as the leg decelerates in preparation for a heel strike. Hip flexion and rotation continue while the knee is fully extended. The trunk and pelvis maintain the support position while the ankle is dorsiflexed and the forefoot supinated prior to heel strike. The hamstrings are also contracting to aid in the deceleration.

The stance phase begins with initial contact or heel strike. Hip flexion is 30 degrees with the knees slightly flexed and the ankle in a neutral position. The pelvis is level and the heel contacts the supporting surface. In the loading response as the sole of the foot contacts the floor, the weight is transported to the limbs. The foot is pronated to adapt to various surfaces and contacts the floor while the ankle is plantar flexed approximately 15 degrees. Hips are flexed and laterally rotate while the knee flexes approximately 15 degrees. Trunk alignment is in a neutral position with the stance leg while the pelvis drops slightly and rotates medially on the swing leg.

The midstance phase or point, beginning when the contralateral limb leaves the ground and ending when the body is directly over the supporting limb, aligns the body over the trunk and pelvis with the level in a neutral rotation. The hip assumes the greatest force with extension to a neutral position. The knee also flexes while the ankle goes from plantar flexion to 10 degrees dorsiflexion while the forefoot is pronated and hindfoot inverted.

The terminal stance (heel-off) is from the midstance to point of contact with the contralateral extremity. The trunk is erect and the hip moves from lateral to medial rotation. The knee is extended and the ankle is in plantar flexion (with heel-off) prior to contact of the opposite foot. In the preswing phase, the initial contact of the contralateral extremity is prior to the toe-off of the reference extremity. The pelvis is level and laterally rotated and the trunk is aligned over the lower extremities. The knee is flexed 35 degrees and plantar flexion of the ankle is approximately 20 degrees to toe-off.

Abnormal Gait

In order to accurately assess difficulties with gait and the accompanying movement problems, it is necessary to observe improper elements of gait to determine specific causes and dysfunctions. Included in Table 8.4 are several examples of gait abnormalities that are commonly seen in school, recreational, and clinical settings (Magee, 1987; Norkin, 1988; Soderberg, 1986). Although this is not a complete list of gait abnormalities, these examples should be helpful in formulating information that is needed to understand movement problems and develop the instructional program.

Detecting Gait Abnormalities

Assessment of gait should occur by observing the specific joint or body segments during the gait cycle (Los Amigos Research and Education Institute, 1993; see Table 8.4). Table 8.5 is based on observation of a child's gait at the Pediatric Exercise and Motor Development Clinic at the University of Georgia, and Figure 8.2 (Range of Motion Summary), Table 8.3 (Gait Terminology), and Table 8.4 (Common Gait Abnormalities).

It should be noted that specific limitations with posture and accompanying gait problems should be documented and determined by the relevant characteristics that contribute to the movement problem. The resulting program planning should specifically address the problem (i.e., balance or strength deficiency) and incorporate it into the program plan. Follow-up assessment and observation can then be utilized to document the effectiveness of the intervention or teaching program.

TABLE 8.4 Common Gait Abnormalities

Gait Abnormalities	Phase	Possible Cause	Characteristics	Assessment
Ataxic	Initial contact	Cerebellum Ataxia and lack of motor control	Poor balance, broad base, exaggerated stagger to movements	Static balance Romberg test for standing posture
		Weakness of dorsiflexor, lack of lower limb proprioception	Foot slap, watches feet while walking, irregular jerky gait	Walking line or beam, foot placement
Gluteus medius (Trendelenburg gait)	Stance	Weakness of gluteus maximus	Excessive lateral tilt or lean to compensate for muscle weakness, bilateral weakness resulting in waddling gait	Evaluate muscle strength or pain in hip
Gluteus maximus	Stance	Weakness of gluteus medius	Lurching or leaning posteriorly, hyperextension at hip	Evaluate muscle strength and pelvic position
Hemiplegic gait	Swing	Weak hip flexors, lack of motor control	Circumduction or lateral movement of entire lower extremity with adduction and internal rotation, affected upper limb may be carried across trunk for stability	Assessment of strength of hip flexors and extensors, range of motion in hip, knee flexion and ankle dorsiflexion
Scissors gait	Swing	Spasticity	Lack of motor control of hip adductor causes knees to move to midline, legs are moved forward by swinging hips	Assess foot placement and control of swinging leg

TABLE 8.4—*Continued*

Gait Abnormalities	Phase	Possible Cause	Characteristics	Assessment
Footdrop or toedrag	Swing	Weakness of dorsiflexor and toe extensor, spasticity in plantar flexors, lack of hip or knee flexion	Weak dorsiflexion of foot does not allow toes to clear the surface, loss of control of dorsiflexors causes higher knee lift to compensate for toedrops resulting in foot slap	Assess strength and range of motion in ankle, hip, and knee
Circumduction	Swing	Weak hip flexors, spasticity	Lateral movement on affected leg to move leg forward abduction, external rotation adduction, and internal rotation	Assess range of motion and strength of hip and knee flexors, ankle dorsiflexors

TABLE 8.5 Observational Analysis of Gait Example

Body Segment	Observation	Direction	Phase	Body Side	Comments
Trunk	Rotation-circumduction	Lateral movement	Swing	Right	Arm adduction and flexion at elbow and wrist, for arm rotated medially
Pelvis	Rotation-circumduction	Lateral movement	Swing	Right	
Hip	Rotation-circumduction	Adduction	Swing	Right	Leg swings outward in a circle (circumduction)
Knee	Reduced flexion	Adduction	Swing	Right	
Ankle	Ankle dorsiflexion	Adduction	Swing	Right	
Feet	Toedrag	Adduction	Swing	Right	Inadequate hip flexion

Cause/Remediation: Neurological dysfunction; assess range of motion and strength in lower extremities

References

Althoff, S. A., S. M. Heyden, and L. D. Robertson. "Posture Screening: A Program that Works." *Journal of Physical Education, Recreation and Dance, 60,* 1988, 20–24.

American Academy of Orthopedic Surgeons. *Joint Motion: Methods of Measuring and Recovery.* Chicago, IL: American Academy of Orthopedic Surgeons, 1975.

Bampton, S. *A Guide to the Visual Examination of Pathological Gait.* Philadelphia: Temple University Rehabilitation Research and Training Center #8, Moss Rehabilitation Hospital, 1979.

Bobath, B. *Adult Hemiplegia: Evaluation and Treatment,* 3rd ed. London: Butterworth-Heinemann Ltd., 1990.

Clark, J. E., and J. Whitall. "Changing Patterns of Locomotion: From Walking to Standing." M. H. Wollacott and A. Shumway-Cook, Eds. *Development of Posture and Gait Across the Lifespan.* Columbia, SC: University of South Carolina Press, 1989.

Gronley, J. K., and J. Perry. "Gait Analysis Techniques." *Observational Gait Analysis.* Downey, CA: Los Amigos Research and Education Institute, Inc., Rancho Los Amigos Medical Center, 1993.

Horvat, M. *Physical Education and Sport for Exceptional Students.* Dubuque, IA: Wm. C. Brown, 1990.

Magee, D. J. *Orthopedic Physical Assessment.* Philadelphia: W. B. Saunders Co., 1987.

Meidaner, J. A. "The Effects of Sitting Positions on Trunk Extension for Children with Motor Impairment." *Pediatric Physical Therapy, 2,* 1990, 11–14.

New York State Department of Education. *The New York Physical Fitness Tests: A Manual for Teachers of Physical Education.* Albany, N.Y.: Department of Education, 1958.

Norkin, C. "Gait Analysis." S. B. O'Sullivan and T. J. Schmitz, Eds. *Physical Rehabilitation: Assessment and Treatment,* 2nd ed. Philadelphia: F. A. Davis, 1988.

Payne, G., and L. D. Issacs. *Human Motor Development: A Lifespan Approach,* 3rd ed. Mountain View, CA: Mayfield Publishing Co., 1995.

Soderberg, G. L. *Kinesiology: Application of Pathological Motion.* Baltimore: Williams and Wilkins, 1986.

Sudgen, D. A., and J. Keogh. *Problems in Movement Skill Development.* Columbia: University of South Carolina Press, 1990.

Thelen, E., B. D. Ulrich, and J. I. Jensen. "The Developmental Origin of Locomotion." M. H. Wollacott and A. Shumway-Cook, Eds. *Development of Posture and Gait Across the Lifespan.* Columbia, SC: University of South Carolina Press, 1989.

Vaughan, C. L., B. L. Davis, and J. C. O'Connor. *Dynamics of Human Gait.* Champaign, IL: Human Kinetics Publishers, 1992.

Vaughan, C. L., B. L. Davis, and J. C. O'Connor. *Gait Analysis Laboratory: An Interactive Book and Software Package.* Champaign, IL: Human Kinetics Publishers, 1992.

CHAPTER 9

Behavior, Leisure, and Play

Preceding chapters have addressed assessments specific to physical and motor fitness development and motor skill acquisition. In the continuing effort to focus on overall development, additional information interrelated with fitness development and skill acquisition should be considered. Each additional information area will provide relevant information regarding capabilities in school, clinical, home-based, and recreational settings. This chapter will focus on specific assessments of behavior (which also includes self-concept and attitudes), leisure, and play as each relate to the overall development of individuals with disabilities.

Behavioral Tests

Assessments of specific behaviors and participation in group activities are often difficult to determine. Measurement of group participation is usually provided through informal tests of behavior including checklists and rating scales. Participation assessments may involve the assessment of social interaction as well as cognitive "style" in the activity setting. Behavioral assessments can provide a meaningful data base for maintaining desirable behaviors and affecting behavior change where change is indicated.

Certain behaviors may interfere with the formal testing process which, in turn, may make behavior test data difficult to interpret. The following guidelines are offered to help ensure that behavior assessment does, indeed, provide an accurate portrayal of the person's behavioral status:

1. The setting must be controlled to define antecedents, behaviors, and consequences.
2. Measurement must include forms of environmental stimulation (e.g., bright lights or loud noises) that are present while the behavior is occurring.

3. Assessment should focus on providing information that can be used to design, implement, and evaluate programs.
4. Assessment should occur in a naturalistic setting.
5. Assessment should be ongoing and self-corrective. Measurement needs to be repeated on a consistent, time-sampling, or probe basis.
6. Assessment must be situation-specific.

Assessing Behavior

The first step in the assessment process is to define the target behavior to determine the extent of its occurrence prior to treatment. The assessment of behavior depends on accurate observation and precise measurement. It is, therefore, important to define precisely the behaviors to be assessed and be prepared to accurately observe and record them. Behavioral assessments may be used to:

1. Screen for behavior problems that interfere with development
2. Define and quantify specific behavior problems
3. Design interventions to address problem behaviors
4. Monitor effects of intervention and withdrawal of reinforcers
5. Probe retention and generalization of behaviors

It is essential to be specific about the targeted behavior and the antecedent or stimulus events that precede the behavior. For example, some behavior may occur before or after a particular event, time of day, in a certain situation, or with another person, with certain foods, medications, or periods of illness (O'Neill et al., 1990).

Behavior assessments can occur in various ways, depending on the number of responses or time intervals. Several types of behavior measurements include (Kazdin, 1980):

1. Frequency—Recording the number of behaviors during a designated time period
2. Response rate—Recording the frequency number of responses divided by the amount of time in the interval
3. Intervals—Recording target behaviors during a specified time rather than by discrete responses that have a beginning and ending point
4. Time-sampling—A variation of interval recording in which observations are conducted for brief periods at different times rather than during a single block of time
5. Duration—Recording the amount of time the response is observed (effective in continuous rather than discrete behaviors)
6. Latency—A duration measure that observes the time lapse between the cue and a response
7. Categorization—Classifying responses according to their occurrence: correct-incorrect, appropriate-inappropriate
8. Group—Recording the number of individuals who perform a specific behavior or response as opposed to individual responses

Formalized Behavior Assessments

Walker Problem Behavior Identification Checklist (WPBIC)

The checklist (Walker, 1983) is a standardized norm-referenced assessment designed to identify preschool or elementary children with possible behavior problems. Although designed for classroom use, the checklist can also be useful in physical activity settings. The WPBIC measures five areas of behavior with 50 items that describe inappropriate behaviors. Behavior score areas include (1) acting out, (2) withdrawal, (3) distractibility, (4) disturbed peer relations, and (5) immaturity. The checklist can be completed in approximately 15 minutes. A sampling of items is as follows:

1. Habitually rejects the school experience through actions or comments
2. Has temper tantrums
3. Does not obey until threatened with punishment
4. Reacts with defiance to instructions or commands
5. Does not engage in group activities
6. Is overactive, restless, or continually shifting body positions
7. Utters nonsense syllables or babbles to himself or herself or does both

The WPBIC was standardized on 500 preschool, 900 primary grade, and 500 intermediate grade children in the Pacific Northwest. Validity information includes data on criterion validity, factorial validity, and item validity. The reported reliability coefficient is .98. The checklist should be supplemented with other behavioral assessment data to provide a picture of motor behavior as well as "acting out" behavior.

Behavior Rating Profile (BRP-2)

The BRP-2 (Brown and Hammill, 1993) is the norm-referenced measure designed to identify possible behavior problems and provide comprehensive assessment of the individual's current behavioral status from grades 1–12. Information is available from four sources: student, teachers, parents, and peers who assess home behavior, school behavior, and interpersonal relationships.

The Student Rating Scale consists of 60 items with 20 related to school behaviors, 20 to home behaviors, and 20 with peer interactions. Students read the items and respond "true" or "false" to statements such as "I have lots of nightmares and bad dreams" or "I often break rules set by my parents." Statements can also be read to the student, and the examiner may explain meanings of words the student does not comprehend.

The Teacher Rating Scale consists of 30 school behavior items which the teacher responds to as "very much like the student," "like the student," "not much like the student," or "not at all like the student." Example behaviors include "doesn't follow class rules" or is "an academic underachiever." An example of the Teacher Rating Scale is included in Table 9.1.

The Parent Rating Scale includes 30 items to which the parent or both parents respond. Example behaviors include "very much like my child," "like my child,"

TABLE 9.1 Section V. The Teacher Rating Scale Items

This Behavior Rating Form contains a list of descriptive words and phrases. Some of these items will describe the referred student quite well. Some will not. What we wish to know is this: Which of these behaviors are you concerned about at this particular time and to what extent do you see them as problems? Take, for example, Item 1, "Is sent to the principal for discipline." If the student frequently is sent to the principal's office, the rater might check the "Very Much Like the Student" space. If the student is sent to the principal's office on an infrequent but regular basis, the rater might check the "Somewhat Like the Student" space. If the student has been sent to the principal's office on rare occasions, a check in the "Not Much Like the Student" space might be appropriate. If the student never has been disciplined by the principal, the "Not At All Like the Student" space would be indicated. These ratings should reflect your perceptions of the student's behavior. Please do not confer with other teachers in completing this form.

The student	Very Much Like the Student	Somewhat Like the Student	Not Much Like the Student	Not At All Like the Student
1. Is sent to the principal for discipline.	☐	☐	☐	☐
2. Is verbally aggressive to teachers or peers.	☐	☐	☐	☐
3. Is disrespectful of others' property rights.	☐	☐	☐	☐
4. Tattles on classmates.	☐	☐	☐	☐
5. Is lazy.	☐	☐	☐	☐
6. Lacks motivation and interest.	☐	☐	☐	☐
7. Disrupts the classroom.	☐	☐	☐	☐
8. Argues with teacher and classmates.	☐	☐	☐	☐
9. Doesn't follow directions.	☐	☐	☐	☐
10. Steals.	☐	☐	☐	☐
11. Has poor personal hygiene habits.	☐	☐	☐	☐
12. Is passive and withdrawing.	☐	☐	☐	☐
13. Says that other children don't like him/her.	☐	☐	☐	☐
14. Can't seem to concentrate in class.	☐	☐	☐	☐
15. Pouts, whines, snivels.	☐	☐	☐	☐

TABLE 9.1—_Continued_

The student . . .	Very Much Like the Student	Somewhat Like the Student	Not Much Like the Student	Not At All Like the Student
16. Is overactive and restless.	☐	☐	☐	☐
17. Is an academic underachiever.	☐	☐	☐	☐
18. Bullies other children.	☐	☐	☐	☐
19. Is self-centered.	☐	☐	☐	☐
20. Does not do homework assignments.	☐	☐	☐	☐
21. Is kept after school.	☐	☐	☐	☐
22. Is avoided by other students in the class.	☐	☐	☐	☐
23. Daydreams.	☐	☐	☐	☐
24. Has unacceptable personal habits.	☐	☐	☐	☐
25. Swears in class.	☐	☐	☐	☐
26. Has nervous habits.	☐	☐	☐	☐
27. Has no friends among classmates.	☐	☐	☐	☐
28. Cheats.	☐	☐	☐	☐
29. Lies to avoid punishment or responsibility.	☐	☐	☐	☐
30. Doesn't follow class rules.	☐	☐	☐	☐
Sum of Marks in Each Column =	____	____	____	____	
Multiply Sum by	× 0	× 1	× 2	× 3	
Add Products	0	+ ____	+ ____	+ ____	**Total Points Scored** = ____

From Brown, L. L., and D. D. Hammill, _Behavior Rating Profile._ Austin, TX: Pro-Ed, 1993.

"not much like my child," or "not at all like my child" to items such as "is verbally aggressive to parents" or "won't share belongings willingly."

The Sociogram or peer portion of the BRP is not a scale or checklist, but a way of providing peer input. Students are asked questions such as, "With which students in your class would you most/least like to work on a school project?" Classmates are then asked to respond to questions that address interpersonal relationships.

Administration time is approximately 15 minutes for each subscale. The BRP was standardized on 1,996 students, 955 teachers, and 1,232 parents from 15 states. Scores are reported in standard scores and percentile ranks. Concurrent validity was established in comparison with other rating scales and found to be consistent. Various group profiles emerged with nondisabled individuals demonstrating the fewest problem behaviors and emotionally disturbed individuals with the highest incidence of problem behaviors. Test-retest reliability scores ranged from 78 percent for a student rating scale to 91 percent for the teacher rating scale.

Functional Analysis of Problem Behavior

The Functional Analysis of Problem Behavior (FAPB) is a practical guide for collecting information on problem behaviors that can be generalized to home-, school-, or community-based settings (O'Neill et al., 1990). Strategies for the functional assessment include:

1. Interviews with the individual or persons who have contact with the individual
2. Observation of individual over an extended period
3. Manipulation of situations that will not result in the target behavior

Components of the FAPB include:

A. Identifying the behavior (e.g., hits self), topography (e.g., head), frequency (e.g., 8–10 episodes), duration (e.g., 3–5 minutes), and intensity (e.g., hard)
B. Identifying ecological events affecting the behavior including medications, medical complications, sleep cycles, eating routines, diet, and tasks and activities during the day
C. Defining events and situations that predict occurrences of the behavior(s) including time of day, setting, social control, or activity
D. Identifying consequences that maintain the behavior, such as the behavior (screaming); what does he or she get (attention) and what does he or she avoid
E. Defining the efficiency of the undesirable behavior, such as (1) amount of physical effort, (2) does behavior result in payoff, (3) delay between behavior and payoff
F. Defining primary methods of communication including signs, gestures, speech, communication boards, extent to which person can follow instructions
G. Identifying events perceived as positive by the person, such as activity reinforcers, outings, attention

H. What Functional Alternative Behaviors are known by the person, such as socially appropriate behaviors, self-pacing the lesson, or a minimal amount of distractions

I. Provide a history of undesirable behaviors, such as behavior (screaming), duration of problem (2–3 years), programs (time-out, extinction), effect (inconsistent)

Although this program does not provide assessment data, it should be useful because of information provided on antecedent events that may cause problem behaviors. Also, the effectiveness as well as the programs heretofore undertaken may be assessed.

Perceived Physical Competence Subscale for Children (PPCSC)

The purpose of the PPCSC (Harter, 1982) is to access a child's perception of physical competence in sports and outdoor games. The PPCSC is one of four subscales from Harter's Perceived Competence Scale for Children (PCSC) which assesses a child's sense of competence across cognitive, social, physical, and general self-worth domains. The PPCSC contains seven items, and the child is asked to indicate which kind of child he or she is more like, based on two alternatives. The child responds "sort of true" or "really true" to physical competence-related questions, with each item scored from 1 (low perceived physical competence) to 4 (high perceived physical competence).

A 40-item PCSC was initially constructed from existing scales and interviews with children. Factor analysis of the responses from children (n = 215) in 3rd–6th grade resulted in development of each subscale. A final version of the PCSC (28 items) was factor analyzed on a new sample of 133 children.

An internal consistency coefficient of .83 was reported for the PPCSC among 341 children, grades 3–6. Test-retest reliability coefficients across three months (n = 208) and nine months (n = 810) were .87 and .80.

Construct validity of the PCSC was supported through factor analysis. Concurrent validity of the PPCSC was supported by teacher ratings of children's actual physical competence in the gymnasium. Discriminant validity was evident in that children (n = 23) selected for sport teams scored higher on the PPCSC than their nonsport team participant classmates (n = 57).

Psychological Skills Inventory for Sports (PSIS)

The PSIS is designed to assess psychological skills consistent with elite performance (Mahoney, Gabriel, and Perkins, 1987). The PSIS (Form R–5) contains 45 items to assess the areas of performance dealing with anxiety, concentration, self-confidence, mental preparation, and team orientation. Individuals are asked to respond to a 5-point Likert scale on such items as: "I sometimes feel intense anxiety while I am actually performing." Internal consistency reliability coefficients of .72 were reported while construct validity was evidenced by comparison of elite athletes with nonelite athletes. Using item analyses on the five subscales, stepwise discriminant and regression analyses were conducted to discriminate between elite and nonelite athletes and cluster analyses. The PSIS has been used with athletes with disabilities and holds potential for providing useful information on psychological profiles of athletes who have disabilities.

Body-Esteem Scale for Children (BES-C)

The purpose of the BES-C is to assess children's evaluations of their bodies (Mendelson and White, 1982). The BES-C contains 20 items designed to reveal how children feel about their appearance and bodies. They respond "yes" or "no" to items such as "I wish I were thinner" and "Kids my own age like my looks." An internal consistency reliability coefficient was reported among 36 children ages 7.5–12 years. Concurrent validity was evident in a correlation coefficient of .67 obtained between scores on the BES-C and scores on the Piers-Harris Children's Self-Concept Scale.

Piers-Harris Children's Self-Concept Scale

This self-concept assessment for grades 3 through 12 measures six factors: (1) behavior, (2) intellectual and school status, (3) physical appearance and attributes, (4) anxiety, (5) popularity, and (6) happiness and satisfaction (Piers and Harris, 1964). The test consists of 80 statements to which the child responds with "yes" or "no" to such items as "I am unpopular" and "I am well behaved in school." Scores range from 1 to 80, with 1 point given for each response that shows good self-concept. Scores are reported in percentiles for each subscale and total score. Validity is based on factor analysis and comparison with the Lipsitt Children's Self-Concept Scale.

Martinek-Zaichkowsky Self-Concept Scale (MZSC)

The MZSC is a functional test to assess self-concept of children in grades 1 through 8, with five factors including (1) satisfaction and happiness, (2) home and family relationships and circumstances, (3) ability in games, recreation, and sports, (4) behavior, and (5) personality traits and emotional tendency (Martinek and Zaichkowsky, 1977). The child/client is presented with 25 pairs of pictures. In each pair, one picture depicts positive self-concept and the other poor self-concept. The person points to the picture that better reveals how he or she feels. Scores range from 1 to 25, with 1 point being given for each picture pointed to that depicts positive self-concept. Validity is based on factor analysis and comparison with the Piers-Harris Children's Self-Concept Scale.

Leisure Recreation Assessments

The ultimate goal of physical activity is to incorporate health and wellness into each person's life. An important extension of this goal is integrating individuals with disabilities into community-based programs that emphasize physical education and recreational activity. Therefore, assessment and programming that include objectives relating to community-based leisure and recreation should not be ignored.

Comprehensive assessment should include all aspects of using community resources, including leisure and recreational skills necessary for successful integration and activity preferences of the individual. While components of leisure and recreation should be assessed and programmed for all ages, there should be increased emphasis on leisure and recreation programming in secondary level programs (ages 12–21). Wehman and Schleien (1981) propose that the following questions be asked before making decisions about assessment and instruction:

Preference—What skills does the child already demonstrate?

Functioning—What are the child's capabilities and educational needs?

Physical characteristics—What physical characteristics does the student have or lack that may interfere with leisure skills development?

Age appropriateness—Are the skills that have been selected for instruction those in which able-bodied peers might also engage?

Access to materials—What is the child's access to materials (e.g., financial resources, transportation)?

Support of home environment—What persons are available in home, neighborhood, or community environments to reinforce leisure skills development?

One type of assessment, leisure skill inventory, can be used to measure an individual's leisure and recreational skill levels. Leisure skill inventories are primarily criterion-referenced instruments, or simple task analyses of leisure skills. Wehman and Schleien (1981) have suggested an example of a task analysis for tossing a Frisbee (see Table 9.2). This behavioral method of assessment provides a measure of entry level performance as well as a continuous record of progress.

The *I CAN* program (Kelly and Wessel, 1990) provides task analysis assessments and curricula for sport activities (team and individual), leisure activities, backyard or neighborhood activities, outdoor activities, and dance. The primary skills package of the *I CAN* program includes assessments and curricula for numerous basic skills genuine to development of sport, leisure, and recreational interests and competencies.

Other methods of leisure assessment include measuring the level of participation in leisure activities, measuring the individual's attention to the activity, appropriateness of behaviors, and levels of social interaction. In order to prepare the individual to make appropriate leisure and recreational choices as an adult, the evaluator may wish to assess the leisure preferences. Knowledge of the individual's activity choices may aid in facilitating motivation, developing the individualized education program, and teaching skills deemed prerequisites for successful leisure experiences. Following are examples of additional leisure assessments.

Recreation Early Development Screening Tool (REDS)

The purpose of the REDS is to assess the developmental level of individuals functioning at or below 1 year of age (Burlingame, 1988). The REDS was developed specifically for use with populations that are mentally retarded or developmentally

TABLE 9.2 Example of a Task Analytic Assessment

Task Analytic Assessment for Tossing a Frisbee

Step	M	T	W	Th	F
1. Extend hand downward toward Frisbee.	+	+	+	+	+
2. Curl fingers underneath Frisbee.	+	+	+	+	+
3. Position thumb on top edge of Frisbee.	+	+	−	+	+
4. Apply inward pressure with fingers and thumb to grasp Frisbee firmly.	−	−	−	+	+
5. Bend at elbow, raising Frisbee to chest.	−	−	−	−	−
6. Hold Frisbee parallel to ground.	−	−	−	−	−
7. Bring Frisbee inward toward nondominant side of body.	−	−	−	−	−
8. Quickly extend elbow outward away from body.	−	−	−	−	−
9. Snap wrist outward and extend fingers to release Frisbee.	−	−	−	−	−
10. Toss Frisbee 2 feet.	−	−	−	−	−
11. Toss Frisbee 3 feet.	−	−	−	−	−
12. Toss Frisbee 4 feet.	−	−	−	−	−
13. Toss Frisbee 5 feet.	−	−	−	−	−

From Wehman, P., and S. Schleien, *Leisure Programs for Handicapped Persons*. Austin, TX: Pro-Ed, 1981.

delayed, and is currently being tested in a number of pediatric hospitals in the United States. The REDS assesses five areas related to leisure: (1) play, (2) fine motor, (3) gross motor, (4) sensory, and (5) social/cognition. Assessment is undertaken to determine the presence or absence of developmental landmarks and to screen for potential developmental problems. For example, observation of play activities at 2–4 months includes the following (Burlingame, 1988):

2–4 MONTHS

1. Does client demonstrate interest in engaging in self-exploratory and/or self-stimulating activities?
2. Do practice games (repeating activities) make up the major part of the client's play (e.g., opening mouth, sticking out tongue in imitation of staff, enjoys peek-a-boo)?
3. Does client seem to enjoy watching his or her hands, engage in simple repetition of body movements (e.g., kicking legs, moving arms in simple patterns) to experience the sensation of his or her body moving?
4. Does client repeat his or her vocal sounds for own pleasure?

Likewise, gross motor activity is assessed by observing the following (Burlingame, 1988):

0–1 MONTH

1. Does client turn head from side-to-side when prone (lying face down); can client lift head momentarily from the bed?

2. Does client's head have a marked head lag when he or she is being pulled from the lying to sitting position?
3. Does client, when prone, tend to assume a flexed position with pelvis high, but knees not under abdomen?
4. Can client maintain his or her head in an upright position when sitting?

2 MONTHS

1. Can client assume a less flexed position when prone—hips flat, legs extended, arms flexed, and head to side?
2. Does client demonstrate only moderate head lag when pulled to sitting position?
3. Does client lift head almost 45 degrees off the floor when in prone position?
4. Does client usually maintain head in an upright position when sitting, but still bobs forward some?

3 MONTHS

1. Is client able to raise head and shoulders from prone position to a 45 to 90 degree angle when on floor?
2. Can client bear weight on his or her forearms when prone on floor?

4 MONTHS

1. Does client demonstrate good head balance when sitting?
2. Can client raise his or her head and chest off a soft surface (e.g., couch) to an angle of 90 degrees?
3. Can client roll from back to side?
4. Is client able to sit erect or propped up?

The child's positive responses are noted on a developmental graph in months for each of five domains: play, fine motor, gross motor, sensory, and social/cognition. Developmental age is noted in each category (for example, play—6 months, gross motor—10 months).

Functional Assessment of Characteristics for Therapeutic Recreation (FACTR)

The Functional Assessment of Characteristics for Therapeutic Recreation (FACTR) is designed to determine basic functional skills and behaviors (Peterson, Dunn, and Carruthers, 1983; Burlingame, 1990, revision). The FACTR, which measures physical, cognitive, and social-emotional functioning, can be used as a screening tool for all populations. Eleven areas, each related to successful leisure functioning, are assessed. Screening is conducted through observation and reviewing medical records. Each item has a list of descriptive statements such as "no difficulty in ambulatory skills" or "uses a wheelchair for ambulation." The tester marks an "X" in front of the descriptive statement that best describes the functional behavior in question. Results of the FACTR enable programming specific to the individual's unique leisure functioning needs.

STILAP

The STILAP (1990) was designed to assess leisure skill acquisition and aid in achieving a balanced leisure lifestyle (Navar and Burlingame, 1990). The individual's leisure skills participation patterns are assessed in 15 leisure functioning areas. Skills assessed are categorized into leisure competency areas. STILAP assessment helps provide bases for leisure decision making and future program involvement in the 15 leisure functioning areas desired. The 15 areas are as follows:

1. Physical Skill That Can Be Done Alone
2. Physical Skill That She/He Can Participate In
3. Physical Skill That Requires the Participation of One or More Additional Persons
4. Activity Dependent on Some Aspect of the Outdoor Environment
5. Physical Skill Not Considered Seasonal
6. Physical Skill With Carryover Opportunity for Later Years
7. Physical Skill With Carryover Opportunity and Vigorous Enough for Cardiovascular Fitness
8. Mental Skill Participated in Alone
9. Mental Skill Requiring One or More Others
10. Appreciation Skill or Interest Area Which Allows for Emotional or Mental Stimulation Through Observation or Passive Response
11. Skill Which Enables Creative Construction of Self-Expression Through Object Manipulation, Sound, or Visual Media
12. Skill Which Enables Enjoyment/Improvement of the Home Environment
13. Physical or Mental Skill Which Enables Participation in a Predominantly Social Situation
14. Leadership and/or Interpersonal Skill Which Enables Community Service
15. Other

The STILAP (1990) assessment tool has two forms. The first form, the Activity Check List (#150A), enables the student/client to indicate type and amount of activity participation. Items are scored by "M" (for much), "S" (for sometimes), and "I" (for interested). "Much" means the individual participates often in the activity and has a sufficient level of self-satisfying participation.

The second form, the Leisure Profile Score Sheet (#150B), is one wherein the therapist tabulates and calculates the individual responses from the Activity Check List (#150A) in each domain area.

The Leisure Diagnostic Battery

The Leisure Diagnostic Battery (LDB) is designed to assess an individual's leisure functioning as described by how an individual feels about his or her leisure experiences (Witt and Ellis, 1990). The LDB comes in separate long and short form versions for adolescents and adults, and includes the following eight components: Perceived Leisure Competency Scale, Perceived Leisure Control Scale, Leisure

Needs Scale, Depth of Involvement in Leisure Scale, Playfulness Scale, Perceived Freedom in Leisure-Total Score, Barriers to Leisure Involvement Scale, Knowledge of Leisure Opportunities Test, and Leisure Preference Inventory. The first five scales can be summed to determine a Perceived Freedom in Leisure score. If the scores of the first five scales indicate problem areas, the remaining subscales are administrated to provide further diagnostic information.

Play

Movement is very important to many aspects of an individual's functional capability. Play is that aspect of development that is interrelated to cognitive as well as social functioning. Although motor assessments have previously been ignored in play-based assessments, there is a growing realization that valuable information on development can be attained through the medium of play. A prevailing belief in early intervention is that children may be appropriately assessed in unstructured contexts such as play (Bagnato and Neisworth, 1991; Greenspan, 1992; Linder, 1993a). The use of unstructured contexts and clinical judgments based on developmental principles provides a multi-method or convergent assessment of children designed to develop a program plan (Bagnato and Neisworth, 1991; Linder, 1993a).

Linder (1993a) refers to this process as Transdiciplinary Play-Based Assessment (TPBA), a natural and functional method of assessment and intervention. Summary information from TPBA is available in the domains of cognitive, social-emotional, communication and language, and sensorimotor development. The process is dynamic and provides input from information gathered from parents as well as other professionals such as therapists, teachers, or early intervention personnel to provide an adequate picture of the child's functioning through the medium of play and various disciplines. For the child with disabilities, the TPBA is designed to provide developmental information that accounts for variations in functioning and capabilities. For example, children with disabilities may possess various temperaments, abilities to process information and master motivation, or various interaction patterns (Linder, 1993a). In order to adequately assess a child and provide a functional evaluation that can lead to an appropriate program plan, the TPBA provides flexibility in testing, a holistic assessment, involvement of parents, natural environments, process information, and a method to plan the intervention (Linder, 1993a,b). Such an approach should be useful to validating behaviors that are observed in the context of play and should provide a more comprehensive understanding of the overall development of children, including those with disabilities. In turn, we may see a shift from more traditional procedures, such as developmental landmarks, to ecological procedures that are specific and functionally appropriate for assessing the strengths and needs of young children (Bagnato and Neisworth, 1991; Greenspan, 1992; Malone and Stoneman, 1990; Simeonson, 1986).

Although the TPBA includes several domains, this section will deal with sensorimotor development (Linder, 1993a). Major categories from this assessment include:

1. General Appearance of Movement
2. Muscle Tone/Strength/Endurance
3. Reactivity to Sensory Input
4. Stationary Positions Used for Play
5. Mobility in Play
6. Other Developmental Achievements
7. Prehension and Manipulation
8. Motor Planning

With the TPBA, observations of the child's movements are made in conjunction with a play facilitator and compared to approximate age ranges for motor skills that are included. The child is observed during play in the following manner (Linder, 1993a):

Playing with toys in a stationary position

Moving from one area to another

Playing with gross motor equipment

Included in Table 9.3 is a sample Sensorimotor Observation Worksheet. By taking a subsection such as 4. (Stationary Positions Used for Play), observations would be gathered on the prone supine, hands/knees, and standing positions. Observations would occur as the child is able to demonstrate these developmental landmarks in the context of play. For example, the sitting position is vital to receiving information about the environment. According to Linder (1993a), team members must decide if the child can sit alone, needs support to sit, and the amount of support that is required. Head control, base of support, and position of the back are all evaluated to determine developmental functioning and restrictions on movement. The child who sits unsupported can then be observed using his or her arms and hands in a play sequence to manipulate objects, or using his or her arms and trunk to maintain postural stability and balance (Linder, 1993a). A summary sheet will accompany the observation guidelines for each domain to rate the child's performance and provide recommendations. The scoring involves a (+) if the child exhibits the skills within the developmental range, or a (–) for a delay in development, deviation from normal patterns, or poor quality of performance (Linder, 1993a). Linder (1993a) also indicates that a (–) might indicate a need to develop skills in an area or reflect a behavior, temperament, or motivational concern that is interfering with the skill. If categories cannot be rated (+ or –) because of limited information available, a (√) is suggested to provide information from another professional, such as a therapist. Other behaviors may be marked not applicable (NA) or not observed (NO), and used at a later stage in the developmental or intervention process. Included in Table 9.4 is a copy of summary sheet instructions from Linder (1993a, p. 57). Each section of the evaluation accommodates the wide variety of functioning in children with and without disabilities. The TPBA is a viable assessment tool to assess the components of

TABLE 9.3 Sensorimotor Observation Worksheet

Name of child: _____ Date of birth: _____ Age: _____

Name of observer: _____ Discipline or job title: _____ Date of assessment: _____

On the following pages, note specific behaviors that document the child's abilities in the sensorimotor categories. Qualitative comments should also be made. The format provided here follows that of the Observation Guidelines for Sensorimotor Development in Transdisciplinary Play-Based Assessment. It may be helpful to refer to the guidelines while completing this form.

I. General Appearance of Movement

A. Physical appearance
  1. Unusual features:

  2. Height and weight appropriate? (*yes or no*)
B. Motor activity
  1. Independent transition to new area? (*yes or no*)
  2. Primary means of movement:

  3. Amount of movement compared to others:

  4. Play positions:

  5. Frequency of each position:

  6. Avoided motor skills:

II. Muscle Tone/Strength/Endurance

A. Features of normal muscle tone
  1. Parallel appearance and movement? (*yes or no*)
  2. Variety of positions? (*yes or no*)
  3. Coordinated when changing position? (*yes or no*)
B. Common factors of unusual muscle tone
  1. Description of behaviors indicating low tone:

    a. Difficulty holding head up? (*yes or no*)
    b. Slumped posture? (*yes or no*)
    c. Wide base of support? (*yes or no*)
    d. Tendency to lock joints? (*yes or no*)
    e. Tendency to lean against supports? (*yes or no*)
    f. Tendency to "W" sit? (*yes or no*)

From Hall, Susan, in T. W. Linder, *Trandisciplinary Play-Based Assessment: A Functional Approach to Working with Young Children*, rev. ed. Paul H. Brookes Publishing Co., P.O. Box 10624, Baltimore, MD 21285-0624. Used with permission.

TABLE 9.4 Directions for Using Summary Sheets

SUMMARY SHEET INSTRUCTIONS

Definitions of scoring criteria:

+ Child demonstrates:
  1. Skill within an appropriate range of development, based on age charts or other references; *and*
  2. typical behavior patterns, based on professional judgment and expertise; *and*
  3. good quality of performance, based on professional judgment and expertise.

− Child demonstrates:
  1. Delay in development based on age charts or other references; *or*
  2. deviation from normal behavior patterns; *or*
  3. poor quality of performance.

√ Insufficient information was obtained. Further evaluation is required.

NA Not applicable due to the age of the child, disability, or other factors.

NO No opportunity to observe, but further evaluation is not recommended.

Procedures:

1. For each of the *Observation Categories* in the left column, indicate strengths the child exhibited within the area.
2. For each of the *Observation Categories* in the left column, indicate whether the child receives a rating of [+], [-], [√], [NA], or [NO].
3. Under the column heading *Justification*, write a brief explanation of why the child received the rating of [–] or [√]. Documentation of reason for [–] rating will assist in the identification of what the child is ready for. Documentation of reason for [√] rating may aid in selection of future assessment procedures.
4. Under the column heading *Things I'm ready for,* identify specific types of activities or developmental processes that the child is ready for in order to progress to higher-level skills.

From Hall, Susan, in T. W. Linder, *Transdisciplinary Play-Based Assessment: A Functional Approach to Working with Young Children,* rev. ed. Paul H. Brookes Publishing Co., P.O. Box 10624, Baltimore, MD 21285-0624. Used with permission.

play and related developmental domains and may be helpful in evaluating the overall functioning of children, as well as developing an appropriate program plan (Linder, 1993b).

Although adapted physical education or therapeutic recreation will not utilize all of these assessment instruments, it is vital to incorporate all aspects of development and functioning into the program plan. With the increasing emphasis on inclusion in home- and community-based programming across the life span, it is important to document appropriate functioning in the domain related to behavior, play, and leisure functioning.

References

Bagnato, S. J., and J. T. Neisworth. *Assessment for Early Intervention: Best Practices for Professionals.* New York: Guilford Press, 1991.

Brown, L. L., and D. D. Hammill. *Behavior Rating Profile.* Austin, TX: Pro-Ed, 1993.

Burlingame, J. *Recreation Early Development Screening Tool.* Ravensdale, WA: Idyll Arbor, Inc., 1988.

Greenspan, S.I. *Infancy and Early Childhood: The Practice of Clinical Assessment and Intervention with Emotional and Developmental Challenges.* Madison, WI: International Universities Press, 1992.

Harter, S. *Perceived Competence Scale for Child Development, 53,* 1982, 87–97.

Kazdin, A.E. *Behavior Modification in Applied Settings.* Homewood, IL: The Dorsey Press, 1980.

Kelly, L., and J.A. Wessel. *I CAN: Primary Skills.* Austin, TX: Pro-Ed, 1990.

Linder, T.W. *Transdisciplinary Play-Based Assessment: A Functional Approach to Working with Young Children,* rev. ed. Baltimore, MD: Paul H. Brookes Publishing Co., 1993a.

Linder, T.W. *Transdisciplinary Play-Based Intervention: Guidelines for Developing Meaningful Curriculum for Young Children.* Baltimore, MD: Paul H. Brookes Publishing Co., 1993b.

Mahoney, M.J., T.J. Gabriel, and T.S. Perkins. "Psychological Skills and Exceptional Athletic Performance." *The Sport Psychologist, 1,* 1987, 181–199.

Malone, D.M., and Z. Stoneman. "Cognitive Play of Mentally Retarded Preschoolers: Observations in the Home and School." *American Journal of Mental Retardation, 94,* 1990, 475–487.

Martinek, T., and L.D. Zaichkowsky. *Manual for the Martinek-Zaichkowsky Self-Concept Scale for Children.* Jacksonville, FL: Psychologists and Educators, Inc., 1977.

Mendelson, B.K., and D.R. White. "Development of Self-Body-Esteem in Overweight Youngsters." *Developmental Psychology, 21,* 1985, 90–96.

Mendelson, B.K., and D.R. White. "Relation Between Body-Esteem and Self-Esteem of Obese and Normal Children." *Perceptual and Motor Skills, 54,* 1982, 899–905.

Navar, N., and J. Burlingame. *State Technical Institute Leisure Activities Project.* Ravensdale, WA: Idyll Arbor, Inc., 1990.

O'Neill, R.E., R.H. Horner, R.W. Albin, K. Storey, and J. Sprague. *Functional Analysis of Problem Behavior: A Practical Assessment Guide.* Sycamore, IL: Sycamore Publishing Co., 1990.

Peterson, S., J. Dunn, and C. Carruthers. *Functional Assessment of Characteristics for Therapeutic Recreation.* Ravensdale, WA: Idyll Arbor, Inc., 1983.

Piers, E., and D. Harris. "Age and Other Correlates of Self-Concept in Children. *Journal of Educational Psychology, 55*(2), 1964, 91–95.

Simeonson, P.J. *Psychology and Developmental Assessment of Special Children.* Boston: Allyn and Bacon, 1986.

Walker, H.M. *Walker Problem Behavior Identification Checklist.* Los Angeles: Western Psychological Services, 1983.

Wehman, P., and S. Schleien. *Leisure Programs for Handicapped Persons.* Austin, TX: Pro-Ed, 1981.

Witt, R., and G. Ellis. *Leisure Diagnostic Battery.* State College, PA: Venture Publishing, 1990.

CHAPTER 10

Translating Assessment into Action: A Team Approach[1]

Information gathered about an individual's performance, motor proficiency, or level of physical fitness can provide a description of overall functional ability. This array of information is of little use, however, unless the data is interpreted correctly and used to develop and implement program plans. The next step, after the assessment data is generated, is to immediately impact on placement and programming decisions for individuals with disabilities. The general purpose of assessment is not to provide a diagnosis but generate useful information to plan and implement appropriate programs that are functional and achievable.

Bricker (1993, p. 12) indicated that assessment, intervention, and evaluation could be divided into the following:

Phase One: Initial assessment

Phase Two: Formulation of individualized education programs (IEP's) or individualized family service plans (IFSP's) (the authors believe this also pertains to recreational service plans [RSP's])

Phase Three: Intervention

Phase Four: Ongoing monitoring and feedback to individualize and modify intervention

Phase Five: Quarterly evaluation of children, families

Phase Six: Annual or semi-annual evaluation of individuals and family progress as well as group progress

The challenge confronting the programming team is to translate the data gathered from the assessment process into action. This includes guidelines for: (1) the

---

[1]Much of the information in this chapter is written in context with the IEP meeting. The authors believe that procedures are similar for the Individualized Family Service Plan (IFSP) and Recreational Service Plan (RSP).

preparation and interpretation of assessment data, (2) the interactions and roles of members of the programming team, (3) the writing of goals and objectives, (4) making decisions about instructional activities, and (5) establishing procedures for monitoring and evaluation of the instructional plan.

Preparation and Interpretation of Assessment Information

If a comprehensive assessment of functional capabilities has been completed, the tester will be faced with data in varying forms. An informal test of behavior may yield data consisting of summaries of observational tallies. A standardized test will yield raw scores, percentiles, and stanines, while a developmental profile may result in developmental ages. A summation of all available data is required to draw conclusions from this "bank" of data that have been gathered and summarized in different forms. In addition, ongoing information from parents, therapists, teachers, and physicians must be utilized to ensure understanding of individual needs and functional capabilities. However, before the data can be used for program planning and instruction, the tester should prepare the data for interpretation.

Preparing the Data

Whether the assessment results are presented verbally or in written form, a systematic picture of the individual's characteristics should be determined. Included in this information are the following assessment components:

1. Demographic data: Include the full name, birthdate, grade placement, address, telephone number, classroom teacher, parent, and case manager (primary special education teacher, if appropriate).
2. Referral data: Include the name of the person who initiated the referral, the referral date, and the reason for referral.
3. Background data: May include information from physicians, therapists, parents, and others concerning the physical, educational, and sociocultural background and status.
4. Observational data noted during assessment: Notes and comments about the individual's behavior during the assessment sessions should be recorded.
5. Test data: All assessment data should be tallied and summarized in raw score form to prepare for further analysis and interpretation.
6. Functional data: Raw scores and observations should be specific to the task or functional skill. If muscular strength is required in the neck and abdominal area to ensure head control and use of a computer, the data should be documented to promote functional development.

A thorough review of the completed response forms should always ensure that the data have been recorded properly. At this point, the evaluator should choose only relevant data that will be specific to program planning and avoid any data that may violate individual privacy (e.g., reading achievement scores, family socioeconomic status).

Summarizing Formal Test Data

Several methods are available to expedite the process of summarizing a vast array of test data in order to describe strengths and needs in a concise form to facilitate both communication and decision making. Informal and formal assessment data of the highest quality should first be summarized as raw scores. Note, however, that raw scores by themselves are of extremely limited value. If a formal, standardized test has been administered, raw scores should be converted to allow comparisons with scores achieved by others in the standardization population. Raw scores may also be converted to derived scores such as age-equivalent scores, grade-equivalent scores, percentiles, standard scores, and stanines. Generally, a tester can convert raw scores to other scores by using tables provided in the test manual. Derived scores include:

1. Age-equivalent scores: Raw scores are translated into the average chronological age (CA) at which the students in the standardization population achieved a particular raw score. For example, Kathy, whose CA is 10.3, achieved an age-equivalent score of 5.11 on a bilateral coordination subtest. Kathy's motor performance on this test was like that of students aged 5 years 11 months, revealing a problem area for a child aged 10.

2. Grade-equivalent scores: Raw scores are translated into the average grade at which students in the standardization population achieved a particular raw score. For example, John, who is at the beginning of third grade, achieved a grade-equivalent score of 1.5 (based on a raw score of 6) on an abdominal strength subtest. This means that the average grade-equivalent score in the standardization group that received a raw score of 6 on the subtest was grade 1.5, indicating grade one and five-tenths.

3. Percentiles: Most standardized tests provide tables for the conversion of raw scores to percentile ranks. A percentile rank indicates the percentage of students in the standardization group that received the same raw score or a lower raw score. For example, if Lisa, age 8, achieved a raw score of 14 in running speed and agility, the corresponding percentile rank in the test norms might be the 35th percentile. This means that a raw score of 14 is equal to or higher than the scores achieved by 35 percent of the standardization group. Lisa obtained a score higher than 35 out of every 100 students in a representative sample of 8-year-olds. Percentile ranks are commonly used in IEP team meetings for reporting test results, because they are fairly easy to calculate and interpret.

4. Standard scores: In standardized tests, raw scores are usually converted to standard scores before further conversions to percentiles and stanines are made. Standard scores provide a scale of scores that can be used for comparisons of all students to whom the test was administered. The mean and the standard deviation are used to calculate standard scores, which are usually presented in the norm tables of the test manual. The mean (X) of a set of scores is the arithmetic average, and is usually presented in motor test manuals for students of different ages. The

standard deviation (SD) of a set of scores describes the variability of the scores. For example, Todd, when compared with his age peers, achieved a standard score of 40 on a motor ability test. Since the mean standard score on this test is 50 and the standard deviation is 10, Todd's score indicates that his performance was one standard deviation below the mean of the norm group for Todd's age.

5. Stanines: Some standardized tests allow the tester to convert raw scores to stanines. Stanines are simply ranges of standard scores. The use of stanines has become increasingly popular in public schools for interpreting and describing formal test results. There are nine stanines, or "standard nines." One advantage in using stanine scores is that collapsing the full range of standard scores into nine categories helps guard against over-interpretation of test data, particularly when differences between students' scores are slight. The conversion of raw scores into stanines is usually provided in tables in the test manual.

Derived scores such as percentiles, standard scores, and stanines provide a means for comparing one individual's raw scores with a "normal distribution" of raw scores. The standardization sample reported in the test manual has raw scores that are distributed normally in a bell-shaped curve. Figure 10.1 shows the relationship of derived scores to the normal distribution.

When a formal, standardized test has been administered and raw scores converted to derived scores, a student's test scores may be plotted on a profile. A test profile provides a visual presentation of an individual's test performance, and can be useful in interpreting test results to parents and other team members. Figure 10.2 presents a sample test profile for a child who was administered the Bruininks-Oseretsky Test of Motor Proficiency. A brief study of a child's test profile allows the tester, team members, and parents to ascertain strengths and weaknesses quickly and aid in program planning. In addition, the profile can be used in conjunction with other assessments to aid in the decision-making process.

Summarizing Informal Test Data

When interviews, observational checklists, and criterion-referenced assessment methods are used, the form of the test data is frequently more qualitative than quantitative. Such methods compare a child to a criterion rather than to scores of age peers. Although informal assessment methods have the advantage of being immediately applicable to the understanding and solution of relevant problems and functional skills, the results must be easy to interpret. Some informal measures do include a criterion for motor performance, but the criteria are subjectively established while other criteria may come from a task analysis of the skill or task.

To assist in summarizing informal test information, we recommend that results be depicted in relation to program goals and objectives. For example, if a certain level of physical fitness is consistent with school and program guidelines, the summary of test information should include whether a specific level of functioning (criterion) has been achieved. If not, program objectives can be developed to meet

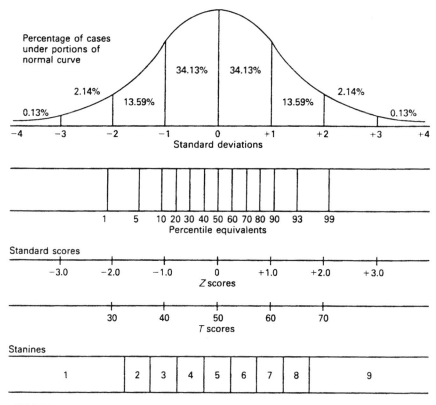

FIGURE 10.1   Relationship of various types of derived scores to the normal curve

program goals and objectives and presented in a summary profile or graph (see Figure 10.2). The levels of mastery for age or grade level may also be recorded, while a clear description of strengths and needs should be readily apparent in an examination of the graph or profile. Since many teachers or clinical personnel have assessment data in varying forms, a summary should be compiled on the student's strengths and needs.

Table 10.1 presents a summary of assessment information from four different assessment instruments. In each case, the information contributed allows the Educational Programming Team to develop a greater understanding of individual needs and functioning. This information can be used for determining the general goals of the Individualized Educational Plan and aids in communicating results and functional capabilities of individuals to parents.

Interpreting Test Results

Once the information from the test has been collected and summarized, the results should be interpreted to suggest program options and implementation strategies

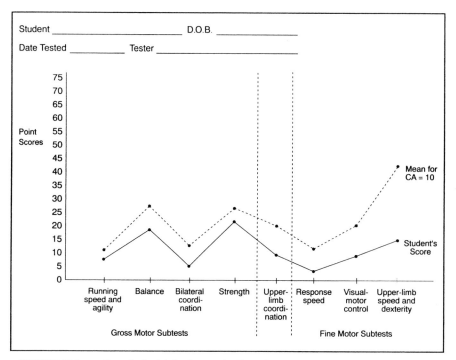

FIGURE 10.2 Sample Bruininks-Oseretsky Test of Motor Proficiency student profile

based on individual needs. At this point, a picture of overall functional capabilities in a variety of areas should be determined to provide the current level of performance in each specific area (i.e., arm strength, static balance, cognition, social interaction). The noted strengths and weaknesses will aid in examining the individuals' needs as well as any relationships to disabilities, or factors that impact on performance and overall physical functioning.

When analyzing the results of data assessment, the evaluator should look for patterns, trends, or flags that can pinpoint potential problem areas. If reliable and valid assessment techniques have been used, consistencies and/or inconsistencies should be noted and checked. For example, if one test revealed deficits in balance but another assessment demonstrated "average" performance, the consistencies should be examined. Another check of reliability and validity may reveal the source of the inconsistencies. Carefully administered tests and assessment methods disclose consistent areas of motor strengths and needs. For example, if one test revealed deficits in upper-limb coordination and if observations of performance demonstrated problems with throwing and catching, the tester can be reasonably

TABLE 10.1 Comprehensive Summary of Areas of Instructional Need

Profile of Instructional Needs from Assessment Data

Client/Child _____
Age _____
Classification _____

	Formalized Test	History/ Developmental Profile	Observation/ Checklist	Criterion-Referenced
Muscular strength & endurance	Persistence of grasping reflex, average in strength for 1 & 10 RPM	Prolonged labor or delivery		
Flexibility	Sit-and-reach scores			
General coordination & perception	Below average on jumping, hopping, object control	Delay in visual perceptual development	Problems with eye-hand coordination	Immature pattern on object control skills
Cardiovascular endurance	Poor in walking test			
Social interaction	At solitary play level in play-based assessment			Withdrawn absences from class. Stands in background: quits
Cognitive skills	Below average on IQ test		Difficulty following game strategies	
Mobility		Delay reaching developmental landmarks		

Recommendations for intervention and placement: _____
_____
_____

confident that these areas represent skill discrepancies. In examining test results for interrelationships, one may determine that balance deficits also coincide with problems in gross agility. Difficulties in locomotor patterns may coexist with problems in an inadequate amount of strength or influence of primitive reflexes as seen in the Figure 10.2 profile. A continuous analysis of text data and input from other team members can be used to note patterns, trends, and inconsistencies among the data before recommendations are made for program planning and instruction.

The evaluator must also study any relationships between potential problem areas and effects of disabilities. For example, an individual with muscular dystrophy will most likely demonstrate deficits in areas of strength, endurance, and locomotor skills in varying degrees, depending on the progress of the disease and age of onset. In this case, we would normally expect to see progressive deterioration of strength or, hopefully, maintenance of functional strength. In contrast, lack of strength and motor control in individuals with cerebral palsy may respond to intervention or erode into the inability to coordinate movements. Likewise, knowledge about learning problems, social interaction or cognitive style can assist in the selection of appropriate instructional strategies based on individual needs.

Next, the tester must explore the degree to which disabilities may influence performance and overall physical functioning. The tester should possess a thorough understanding of the individual's strengths and difficulties as well as the current environment. Several factors that should be considered may include the following:

1. Severity of performance deficits
2. Areas of special educational needs
3. Goals and objectives for motor skill and fitness
4. Expectations for physical functioning outside the school
5. Functional skills for home, work, and leisure settings

Severity of Performance Deficits

The severity of the deficit in performance should be noted and compared by age and/or grade expectations. Standardized tests provide percentile ranks, stanines, and standard scores to facilitate interpretation. One or more standard deviations below the mean, stanine scores of 1, 2, or 3, and percentile ranks of below 16, may all indicate below average performance. Scores closer to the mean (e.g., only 1 or less standard deviations from the mean) indicate potential problems but to a milder degree. These deficits are not severe and may respond to interventions to achieve peer group expectations. Individuals with discrepancies more than 2 standard deviations from the mean in age group expectations may require specialized placement and/or supplementary services to meet their educational goals.

Placement and needs are not always directly linked to numerical ranks. Individuals with functional losses may not fall at a certain rank or level, yet require adequate assessments of their capabilities to offset potential problems that interfere with overall functioning.

When informal assessments are being interpreted, decisions about the severity of discrepancies is more complex. When an individual's performance has been measured against a criterion and does not meet the expected criterion, it is essential to analyze the severity of the discrepancy, individual performance, and the criterion. For example, evaluating performance on a balancing task may be limited by sensory impairment, neurological dysfunction, or poor strength development. Questions should be asked to determine the balance variations in the assessment process. For example:

1. What level of balance should be expected given the age, grade level, and disability, and is it functional?
2. Does the individual possess a sufficient level of strength to complete the task?
3. What complicating factors, such as visual impairment, and ataxia, are present that affect this task?

Special Education Areas of Need

While analyzing the results of the assessment, the tester should note areas that require intervention. An individual with numerous deficits will require more specific intervention than will an individual with difficulties in one area. One individual with below average physical fitness may not require an intensive program, as compared to the individual with general coordination, movement control, low fitness, and communication difficulties. Although special assistance may be needed to improve fitness levels, programming can be implemented within the regular class, at home, or in some combination. In contrast, the other individual may require an extensive program in school in conjunction with the teacher, therapist (speech and physical), and the adapted physical education teacher. Depending on the severity of the difficulties, the program may occur through an adapted specialized class as a training supplement, therapy, or a home-based program. The proposed interventions to meet an individual's needs will be implemented after analyzing the severity and scope of the individual's problem areas, as well as the availability of program services.

Skill and Fitness Goals and Objectives

The expectation for motor skill and fitness levels needed for successful performance in any given setting should also be carefully considered in conjunction with the goals and objectives of the program. For example, an eighth grade class curriculum is based on prerequisite skills for volleyball and soccer, but assessment reveals that the child with a disability exhibits serious difficulties in those prerequisite skills. The tester can be reasonably confident in predicting that the child will struggle with those skills in the regular class, necessitating an individualized program to provide special instruction in prerequisite skill areas. In contrast, for an individual with a lower limb disability, it may be more appropriate to be concerned with fitness skills that allow the individual to function in the school environment or participate in community recreational activities that are consistent with goals for the school.

Expectations for Physical Functioning

Another consideration when interpreting assessment results is the expectations of children for physical functioning in environments outside the school. Expectations for infants and young children would be for ambulation, appropriate play skills, and functioning in leisure and family settings. Older individuals require preparation for transition from school to home settings, community-based recreational programs, and preparing for work-related and vocational skills (Croce and Horvat, 1992; Zetts, Horvat, and Langone, in review). Recognized levels of physical functioning that are appropriate for program planning goals and objectives include:

1. Physical Functioning Level I—nonambulatory, simple upper-body skills such as reach, grasp, trunk control, and head control
2. Physical Functioning Level II—rudimentary locomotion such as creep, crawl, cruise, stand; basic object manipulation such as grasp, release, throw, push, pull; basic body awareness; motor skills for personal care such as feeding, toileting, and dressing, and righting reflexes
3. Physical Functioning Level III—functional patterns of fundamental motor skills such as walk, run, vertical jump, up and down stairs, overhand throw, underhand throw, low to average levels of physical fitness; basic body awareness and body management; participation in playground activities
4. Physical Functioning Level IV—mature patterns in some fundamental skills of locomotion and object control, good static and dynamic balance; average levels of fitness; may participate in intramural activities or sports or community recreational, vocational, or family activities

Team Decision Making

When results from individualized assessment are used in an Individualized Educational Plan (IEP), Individualized Family Service Plan (IFSP) meeting, or Recreational Service Plan (RSP), the results should be shared and discussed with a team of parents and professionals who cooperate to make the best possible programmatic decisions. Teachers, including adapted physical education/therapeutic recreation personnel, should provide valuable contributions to the IEP/IFSP/RSP planning meeting, and attempt to attend all meetings or at least provide a written summary of the physical, motor, and/or leisure capabilities of individuals with disabilities.

The Program Planning Meeting

The purposes of the program planning meeting are to discuss the results of assessment procedures to determine eligibility and special services, and to design an appropriate educational or services plan. To meet state regulations, this IEP meeting must usually take place within 30 calendar days of a determination that the student has a disability and is in need of special services. A completed IEP must be in place before the services are to be delivered, and must be implemented as soon as possible after the meeting. After the initial meeting, an IEP meeting is held annually to reexamine and revise the program. This should also be the case for the IFSP/RSP following the six phases espoused by Bricker (1993).

Case Manager

When an individual has been referred for special education assessment for the first time, a *case manager* is assigned to facilitate ongoing communication with other team members about the status of due process procedures. Usually, the case manager is someone specially trained in the area of the child's primary disability. An adapted education teacher will generally be the case manager only for those students whose primary disability is a physical impairment that interferes solely with physical education. The case manager has the primary responsibility for notifying all team members of the time and place of the planning meeting, as well as the following concerns:

1. Due date for completed assessments
2. Time and place of the meeting
3. Information needed for parents
4. Written parental permission for assessment and implementation of the program plan
5. Names of other team members

Participants in the Program Planning Meeting

The program planning team is composed of representatives from various allied professions. For the IEP the team may include: (a) the school nurse, (b) a psychologist, (c) regular and special education teachers, (d) a speech and language clinician, (e) a physical and/or occupational therapist, (f) a physician, and (g) other special education or related service personnel. The participants at the program planning conference must include: (a) a representative from the school to supervise the meeting (e.g., principal), (b) the student's teacher or teachers, (c) one or both parents or guardians, (d) the child, if appropriate, and (e) a team member who performed the assessment (e.g., adapted physical education teacher or therapeutic recreation specialist).

Classroom Teacher

The child's assigned classroom teacher should be in attendance at the IEP meeting to share observations of the child's physical functioning in the classroom and the entire school environment. The teacher may provide valuable insights into the personality, attending behavior, social skills, and work habits of students.

Physical Education Teacher

At a meeting where results of a developmental/adapted physical education assessment are to be discussed, the child's regular physical education teacher should be present. During the meeting, the physical education teacher will share observations of the student's participation in class as well as any assessment information. Information related to scheduling should be provided to assist in developing goals and objectives that are consistent with class participation in the regular class. In addition, the discussions at the program planning meeting may provide the physical education teacher with more information about the child's strengths, needs, and unique characteristics. If this teacher can attend this conference, it will aid in developing a greater awareness of children with disabilities and contribute to the insights of other professionals.

Therapist

In some instances, physical and/or occupational therapists may participate in the IEP meeting. Information regarding physical functioning, such as range of motion, muscle tone, muscle strength, reflexes, and suggestions regarding the use of braces or other adaptive equipment, can be useful for teachers as well as give suggestions or guidelines for transfers, positioning, and handling in various orthopedic or multihandicaps.

An occupational therapist shares results of an evaluation of a child's functional performance on reflexes, fine motor skills, sensorimotor functioning, and self-help skills. Since many of the functions overlap, it is essential for physical therapy, occupational therapy, therapeutic recreation, and adapted physical education to interact closely in a professional manner to provide the best possible programmatic emphasis without regarding roles.

Special Education Teachers

Special education personnel provide special educational services for the student. In addition to the possibility of being appointed case manager, they bring essential information to the other team members on the disability, learning style, attention span, effective development, behavior potential, motivators, and reinforcers.

Recreational Therapist

The recreational therapist (RT) is generally not available in a school setting. However, the services of the RT in a community-based recreational setting can contribute to the social, emotional, and physical functioning of individuals with disabilities.

A recreational therapist can provide leisure assessments for play and recreation and integration into community activities that can be lined to program objectives. In addition, RT's can provide opportunities for sports participation and a continuum of services from the regular educational setting as well as providing much of the information for the RSP.

Parent and Child

The parent or parents (or the guardians) are required to attend the IEP meeting. If they are not in attendance, the program may not be initiated without their written permission.

Parents can offer interesting and helpful information about their child at the IEP or Individualized Family Service Plan meeting. They also can work closely with therapeutic recreational personnel to determine the RSP and activities outside the school in a recreational or play setting. Descriptions of the child's play behavior in the home, the yard, and recreational settings provide a clearer picture of the child's physical functioning in the natural living environment. A child who resides in a small, one-bedroom high-rise apartment may have less opportunity for gross motor play than the child living in a ranch style house in a sprawling suburban neighborhood. Being aware of physical activity levels available at home can aid in determining program goals and objectives. The program planning meeting also is an opportunity to provide suggestions for enhancing play or overall development through a home-based program.

When appropriate, the child may participate in his or her own program planning meeting. Children in intermediate through secondary grade levels who have the ability to participate in the decision-making process should attend program planning meetings and can provide insight into his or her interests and needs in physical education. Children who assist in setting goals and objectives may also be highly motivated to participate in the developmental/adapted physical education program and to monitor their own progress.

The Principal and Others

Federal law mandates (IDEA, 1990) that a representative from the local education agency (LEA) participate in and supervise the program planning meeting. The representative is usually the building principal, although an assistant principal, guidance counselor, or teacher can sometimes be designated instead. The principal's role at the program planning meeting is to guide the decision-making process and to be a liaison between school and parents. The principal can offer a unique perspective on the overall administration and management of the proposed individualized program, as well as assist in the communication process and general operation of the meeting.

For some children, there may be additional participants at the program planning meeting. Family physicians, medical specialists, and child advocates sometimes attend. Only persons who have assessment results to present or contributions to make toward the development of the program should participate in the conference.

Communication during Program Planning Meetings

If professionals are well prepared and knowledgeable about assessment results, the key to productive decision making is effective communication among team members. Effective communication requires sharing and discussing the assessment data to portray an adequate picture of the individual. The development of an appropriate instruction program is the intent of the program planning conference. This goal cannot be accomplished without communication and collaborative efforts among team members (without regard to role or issues of responsibility), whether the program is ultimately implemented in the school, home, or community setting.

Reviewing Rights

Often overlooked in the development of the IEP are the specific due process rights of parents. While federal mandates guarantee parental rights in the education of children with disabilities, most states have more specific regulations delineating step-by-step due process procedures. At the beginning of each IEP conference, the case manager or designated staff member should briefly explain and review the rights and due process system for the parents. This review is not intended to be a legal "reading of the rights" activity, but rather a reminder to everyone present that the parent or guardian has an equal partnership role in the decision-making process.

Sharing Results

Each team member who conducted an assessment must present their findings at the program planning conference. Since a program planning conference usually takes place in a limited amount of time, some general suggestions for efficient reporting follow.

General Procedure Used

The report should be presented by briefly reviewing the assessment procedure. If a standardized fitness test was administered, a brief description of the reason fitness was measured and the instrument or method used should be given. If no standardized tests were used, explain the uniqueness of the child's needs and why informal methods were selected instead.

Clarity

Titles of subtests and terminology may sound like jargon to other team members or parents. When reporting test results, explain briefly the meaning of the term and provide examples to team members or parents.

Reporting Ranges

Instead of reporting specific scores, the results of an assessment should be explained descriptively. For example, rather than reporting a score of 17 on balance was achieved, it is more understandable to report that the individual's balance skill level was below average for her age or at the 10th percentile. In addition, it should be specific to functional skill development. For example, the low score on balance is one of the major reasons the child has difficulty walking up stairs. McLoughlin and Lewis (1981) proposed a five-level system for reporting assessment results.

1. Above average: more than 2 standard deviations above the mean
2. High average: from 1 to 2 standard deviations above the mean
3. Average: within 1 standard deviation above or below the mean
4. Low average: from 1 to 2 standard deviations below the mean
5. Below average: more than 2 standard deviations below the mean

When using this system, the reporter can simply indicate the desired scores, or age equivalents, with the corresponding levels listed above, if desired. Each statement of assessment results should be a statement about the child's current level of performance. As a current skill status is explained, the above system can be used to report strengths as well as weaknesses. When motor performance in one area seems to be related to performance in another area, indicate the relationship.

Recommendations

While reporting assessment results, it is advisable to postpone making recommendations until later in the conference. As results are summarized and explained, emphasize clearly the areas of strengths and difficulties. It is both professional and wise to listen to the reports of other team members, to ask relevant questions, and to answer the questions that others may have before making recommendations.

Listening to Team Members

Although the role of the adapted physical education teacher may appear to be one of reporting assessment results and making recommendations, assuming the role of listener is equally important. Parents can provide interesting insights into the child's physical functional and motor behavior, while personnel such as the school nurse may well have worthwhile observations on effects of medication. Everyone present at the program planning conference plays an important role in shaping the program development process, and information gleaned from a variety of sources allows for informed programming decisions.

Writing the Program Plan

According to federal guidelines concerning the contents of the program plan, it is essential to include the following:

1. Statement of the child's present levels of educational performance
2. Statement of annual goals, including short-term objectives
3. Statement of the specific educational and related services to be provided to the child, and the extent to which the child will be able to participate in regular educational programs
4. Projected dates for initiation of services and anticipated duration of services
5. Appropriate objective criteria, evaluation procedures, and schedules for determining on at least an annual basis whether the objectives are being achieved

Current Level of Performance

A brief statement concerning the current level of performance should be developed to indicate general areas of needs and functional capabilities. Usually, this statement is incorporated with information from other team members concerning the present state of the individual's capabilities. This information is specific to developing the IEP as well as the IFSP and RSP.

Annual Goals

Annual goals should represent recommendations for instruction within the instructional period or academic year. Since the goals are broad-based generalizations, they may vary according to the individual capabilities, age, areas of need, input from parents, and expectations with the regular instructional setting. Although they may vary by individual or setting where the instruction will occur (home, community) they should be based on results of the assessment data and current level of functioning.

Fitness Goals

Physical fitness is a goal for all individuals, beginning with preschool and primary grade children who require sufficient levels of strength and endurance to stand, ambulate, and ascend and descend stairs as well as perform some motor skills that require sufficient fitness such as jumping. Fitness becomes a more crucial goal for intermediate and secondary grades, as individuals are required to ambulate, perform activities for long periods of time, and begin vocational skills training. It is essential that a determination of the individual's functioning be clearly documented to determine if low levels of fitness are affecting their capabilities, or in the case of high school-aged individuals, what type of fitness is required for transition into community recreation or in a work-performance situation (Zetts, Horvat, and Langone, in review). Examples of annual physical fitness goals are:

1. John will improve abdominal strength.
2. John will improve cardiovascular endurance by walking consistently for 30 minutes.
3. John will increase his upper body strength by 20 percent.
4. John will improve overall flexibility.

Locomotor Skill Goals

If it is determined that a component of fitness is lacking, appropriate goals can be initiated in that area. Some children may have needs in the development of motor skills that should be addressed. For example, if delays in motor skills are evident from the assessment data that interfere with play-based behaviors, and subsequent parental observations substantiate that locomotor skills are delayed, goals may be written for improving locomotor skills (Horvat, Malone, and Deener, 1993). Sample annual goals for locomotor skills are:

1. Beth will demonstrate a mature creeping pattern for 8 to 10 feet.
2. Beth will walk unassisted and maintain balance for 10 steps.
3. Beth will demonstrate arm opposition while walking.

Locomotor skill goals include creeping, crawling, walking, running, vertical jumping, horizontal jumping, hopping, galloping, skipping, sliding, and leaning. Specially designed locomotion goals may include propelling a wheelchair or walking with canes or other assistive devices. In addition, infants and toddlers delayed in achieving developmental milestones may require motor goals to develop appropriate play skills (Horvat et al., 1993).

Goals for Object Control Skills

The ability to manipulate objects is important from preschool through secondary grades. Object control skills for infants are needed to receive adequate sensory information by manipulating or exchanging objects, as well as serving as sensory lures for infants to reach and initiate crawling movements (Horvat et al., 1993). For older children, play, sports, and recreational activities require grasping, releasing, and controlling objects. Each of these activities is important in school, home, and community settings. In addition many self-help skills require identical prerequisite skills for functional needs such as dressing. Sample annual goals for object control skills are:

1. Jason will demonstrate a mature overhand throw with distance (30 feet) and accuracy (10-foot diameter target).
2. Jason will grasp a 4-inch Nerf ball 9 to 10 times.
3. Jason will move object from one hand to another 4 to 5 times.
4. Jason will initiate movements to a ball and grasp the object 4 to 5 times.

Object control skill goals for preschool-age children for play and development may include push, pull, reach, exchange, manipulate, grasp, release, and an underhand roll (Fewell, 1991; Linder, 1993b). Elementary level skills include overhand throw, catch, kick, batting, underhand strike, and ball bounce. Object control skills at secondary levels include dribbling, shooting baskets, chest pass, one-hand catch, tennis serve, tennis volley, volleyball serve and volley, soccer kicks, soccer dribbling, golf swing, shuffleboard push, racquetball swing, and bowling swing. Other object control skills may include buttoning, zippering, tieing, writing, and typing on a computer.

Body Management Goals

Several motor ability and developmental profiles include subtests that measure the components of body management, including balance and awareness of body parts, laterally and directionally. Goals for improving balance are appropriate for children and infants who should maintain an upright position, to individuals requiring balance to ski or jump rope at preschool through secondary levels. In order to generalize the results of test items that evaluate balance into meaningful instructional goals and activities, the following examples may include:

1. Mary will maintain a 1-foot balance for 10 seconds.
2. Mary will balance on 3 parts of her body for 10 seconds.
3. Mary will walk heel-to-toe for 6 consecutive steps following a 2-inch tape line.
4. Mary will maintain a tripod position for 10 seconds.

Tests that address equilibrium, vestibular system function, or righting reflexes are in essence purporting to measure various factors in the balance domain in either static (maintaining balance while stationary) or dynamic (maintaining balance while moving) positions.

Other body management goals focus on the areas of agility, spatial direction, body actions, body awareness, and spatial relations. Examples of body management goals are:

1. Dan will identify basic body parts on request (body awareness).
2. Dan will move on request according to the directions forward, backward, sideways, up, down, over, and under (spatial direction).

3. Dan will demonstrate the body actions of twist, turn, bend, straighten, and reach on request (body actions).
4. Dan will participate in a large-group physical activity and maintain his own self space while respecting the space of others. He will not bump into other children or objects as he moves across the playground (spatial relations).

Goals for Social Interaction

An often overlooked area in development is the social interaction that is necessary for successful participation in physical education and leisure settings. Although the social domain persuant to federal mandates is not considered a part of the instructional process, it is critical to the overall developmental process. In the very basic stages of play development, lack of social interaction interferes with developing cooperation, communication, and appropriate interactions with peers (Bailey and Wolery, 1989; Horvat et al., 1993). Difficulties with social skills generally are not assessed in most standardized physical education tests. Social participation can be assessed by recording observed social behaviors and interactions in a naturalistic play, home-based or instructional setting. In addition, inappropriate social responses can interfere with instruction and affect learning (Malone and Stoneman, 1990). Further, children deprived of social interaction opportunities may also demonstrate deficits in physical and motor skill proficiency. When social problems are clearly interfering with safe and successful participation in physical activity, annual social skill goals should be written into the IEP. Sample annual goals in the social domain are:

1. Joe will cooperate with others by taking turns and sharing his toys.
2. Joe will play with 1 or 2 other children in a cooperative setting.
3. Joe will respect play equipment by using it properly and safely.
4. Joe will participate in group games by congratulating the opposing team when his team loses.
5. Joe will attend and follow directions in the activity setting.

Goals in the social domain may also interact directly with other annual goals, such as appropriate behaviors, and may be directly related to how much the individual learns and develops. When appropriate, goals should be written to include behaviors that are general to home and recreational settings. For example, goals in the social domain such as taking turns, decreasing inappropriate behaviors, respecting the performance of others, using equipment properly, and attending and interacting properly are all consistent in instructional and home-based settings.

Other Annual Goals

Annual goals may be written for any problem area in the developmental domain, and should be broad enough to address the individual needs category of skills for which specific objects are written. Since the IEP is in part a communication tool for the school and the child's parents, annual goals should be written clearly to address all input from team members.

Instructional Objectives and Criteria

Once the annual goals are established delineating major areas of need for individualized intervention, specific instructional objectives should be developed for each annual goal area. Instructional, short-term objectives are statements about specific physical education skills to be developed to attain a particular annual goal. For example:

1. *Goal:* To develop a mature running pattern
   Objectives:
   a. Given 1 minute, a running course of at least 50 yards, and the verbal cue, "Run until I say stop," the child will demonstrate running with arms in opposition to legs 90 percent of the time.
   b. Given 1 minute, a running course of at least 50 yards, and the verbal cue, "Run until I say stop," the child will demonstrate running with heel-toe placement 95 percent of the time.
2. *Goal:* To improve abdominal strength
   Objectives:
   a. Given 30 seconds, the child will demonstrate 20 curl-ups with knees bent and hands behind head.
   b. Given 20 seconds, the child will demonstrate continuous V kicks 1 inch from floor while balanced on seat and elbows.
3. *Goal:* To demonstrate a functional vertical jump
   Objectives:
   a. Given a 3-foot square, the child will demonstrate 9 or 10 vertical jumps with feet together, full arm swing, and maintaining balance when landing.

Clarity will aid in communicating the objectives to parents, team members, and the children, and will also provide clear and specific guidelines for instruction as well as evaluating progress and achievement.

In order to develop appropriate instructional objectives that are specific to annual goals, the following guidelines should be observed:

1. State the task or skill in behavioral terms, including positioning (e.g., 30-to-40 degree curl-ups with bent knees and hands clasped accross the chest).
2. Describe the instructional cues, environmental boundaries, time limits, and equipment.
3. State the criteria for attainment, the standard against which the individual will be measured (e.g., 9 of 10 trials).

Service Delivery

When assessment is completed and individual needs identified, the means for meeting the instructional activities must be decided. The program should be determined by individual needs in the least restrictive environment rather than defining the needs to accommodate the available program facilities. The convenience of facilities, equipment, and programs too often dictate how services are delivered.

Least Restrictive Environment

The individual's program should be delivered in the least restrictive environment to meet documented needs. Aufsesser (1991) developed a range of adapted physical education services that range from traditional specialized classes to home- and community-based interaction. Recently, the focus on inclusion has seen variable placements in regular and specialized settings. For many students, the provision of physical education, recreation, or home-based services should be in the least restrictive setting and in a manner conducive to the individual's needs that need to be explored. Modifications of program plans, aids, and consultation with other teachers and support services may fulfill the needs of many individuals for safe and successful instruction in school and community settings. For individuals with severe disabilities, individualized programs conducted on a one-to-one or small-group basis may be more appropriate as the least restrictive environment. The primary concern should be on individual needs and expectations. By using a functionally based curriculum we can implement program plans to acquire age group and developmental skills in preschool and the primary grades as well as community and recreational settings. As individuals progress through the school years, the emphases may change to daily living, transitional skill and work-related skill, and fitness or leisure development aimed previously at community participation. At each level we must be sensitive to the individual's needs and evaluate his or her capabilities based on goals for the situation.

Sample Case Studies

Included in Appendix A are several sample cases that provide results from test data. Analyze the results and prepare a placement recommendation, goals, objectives, and a sample program plan.

References

Aufsesser, P. M. "Mainstreaming and Least Restrictive Enviroment: How Do They Differ?" *Palaestra, 4,* 1991, 31–34.

Bailey, D. B., and M. Wolery. *Assessing Infants and Preschoolers with Handicaps.* Columbus, OH: Charles E. Merrill Publishing Co., 1989.

Bricker, D. *AEPS: Measurement for Birth to Three Years* (Vol. 1). Baltimore, MD: Paul H. Brookes Publishing Co., 1993.

Croce, R., and M. Horvat. "Effects of Reinforcement-Based Exercise on Fitness and Work Productivity in Adults with Mental Retardation." *Adapted Physical Activity Quarterly, 9*(2), 1992, 148–178.

Fewell, R. "Trends in the Assessment of Infants and Toddlers with Disabilities." *Exceptional Children, 58*(2), 1991, 166–173.

Horvat, M., D. M. Malone, and T. Deener. "Educational Play: Preschool Children with Disabilities." S. Grosse and D. Thompson, Eds. *Play and Recreation for Individuals with Disabilities: Practical Pointers.* Reston, VA: AAHPERD, 1993, 58–66.

Public Law 101–476. (1990, October 30). *Individuals with Disabilities Education Act Amendments of 1990*, 1103–1151.

Linder, T. W. *Transdisciplinary Play-Based Assessment,* rev. ed. Baltimore, MD: Paul H. Brookes Publishing Co., 1993a.

Linder, T. W. *Transdisciplinary Play-Based Intervention.* Baltimore, MD: Paul H. Brookes Publishing Co., 1993b.

Malone, D. M., and Z. Stoneman. "Cognitive Play of Mentally Retarded Preschool Children: Observation in the Home and School." *American Journal of Mental Retardation, 94,* 1990, 475–487.

McLoughlin, J. A., and R. B. Lewis. *Assessing Special Students.* Columbus, OH: Charles E. Merrill, 1981.

Zetts, R., M. Horvat, and J. Langone. (In review.) Effects of a community-based strength training program on fitness and work productivity in high school students with mental retardation. Submitted for publication.

Case Studies

CASE 1

NAME: Len Charles
SCHOOL: Bulldog Elementary
GRADE: First
AGE: 7–2
DOB: 9/17/86
DATE OF EXAMINATION: 11/19/93

Test Information

WISC-R: Verbal IQ = 40
                Performance IQ = 110 (MA = 7–8)
                Full Scale = 65
Leiter: MA—9–6
VMI: Age equivalent = 9–4
TOLD: Picture Vocabulary = 5–1 (Language age)
                Oral Vocabulary = 4–2
                Grammatic Understanding = 4–0
                Sentence Imitation = 3–6
                Grammatic Completion = 4–0

NOTE: Delayed 3–10 seconds between the examiner's verbal stimulus and response. Silently looked at the examiner during this period or repeated the word several times.

Auditory Screening Evaluation: Hears all frequencies at 20 decibels. This indicates that hearing is within the normal range.

EEG Abnormal: The EEG shows abnormal activity in the left hemisphere, temporal lobe.

Behavioral Information

Len has difficulty following directions. His teachers are convinced that he is intentionally noncompliant. He looks at the adult when given a direction but seldom follows through with a request. He will follow directions when given in a slow, stern voice or if repeated. At times, Len perseverates on selected words of a direction or statement, repeating them several times.

Len isolates himself in the classroom, usually choosing an art or puzzle activity during free time. He is not active outside nor participates with other children.

Language and Speech

Len's language development is delayed. He is difficult to understand because of poor syntax and articulation. He often pauses when speaking, appearing to seek the next word.

Academic Skills

Len's reading skills are poor and he has difficulty reading phonetically. He cannot discriminate between short vowel sounds. His blending skills are poor and he has difficulty separating words into components. Spelling is a problem.

Len's fine motor skills are excellent. He often draws pictures and can form all numbers and letters correctly.

Bruininks-Oseretsky Test of Motor Proficiency

Subtest	Point Score		Age
	Maximum	Subject's	
Running speed and agility	15	8	6–4
Balance	32	10	4–8
Bilateral coordination	20	5	5–11
Strength	42	5	4–11
Gross motor composite	[28]		

CASE 2

NAME:	Teresa Burt
SCHOOL:	Bulldog Elementary
GRADE:	First
AGE:	7–0
DOB:	10/21/86
DATE OF EXAMINATION:	10/27–28/93

Tests Administered

Battelle Developmental Inventory
Peabody Picture Vocabulary Test
Koontz Child Development Program
Vulpe Assessment Battery
Vineland Adaptive Behavior Scale
Columbia Mental Maturity Scale

Reason for Referral

Teresa was referred for psychological evaluation due to the three-year reevaluation requirement for students in special education programs. Teresa is currently enrolled in the severe mental impairments class.

Background Information

Teresa is currently on Phenobarbitol for seizure activity. She has cerebral palsy which limits her physically. She has limited motor control for expressive speech and does not walk at this time. She is unable to manipulate a pencil with much success. Teresa appears very alert and highly interested in her surroundings. According to the 10/90 evaluation, she has better vision in her right eye and her left eye frequently wanders. Teresa's teacher describes her as being stubborn at times and not always wanting to put forth effort. She learns things quickly as noted from last spring's annual review. On the Brigance, general knowledge was approximately at the 4-year level. Teresa is very aware of time concepts such as yesterday, today, and tomorrow. Academically, Teresa is working on kindergarten level skills. Her favorite color is purple. Teresa weighed 4 lb, 8 oz at birth. She was born eight months into the pregnancy due to hemorrhaging. Teresa has cerebral palsy due to a lack of oxygen at birth.

Previous Test Results

11/19/93	Hearing Screening	Passed
11/19/93	Vision Screening	Failed
2/6/94	Vision examination—Better vision in right eye. Follows light and hand movements. Cannot state whether she is legally blind.	

10/90   Bayley Scales of Infant Development

Area	Age Equivalent
Gross Motor	9 months
Fine Motor	14 months
Social	10 months
Receptive Language	14 months
Expressive Language	8 months

Test Behavior

During the evaluation, Teresa was cooperative at times and stubborn at other times. She enjoyed the individual attention and loved to work. She was always neatly groomed and appeared in good health. Teresa was very attentive for long periods of time. She worked willingly and spoke to me on the second day. Teresa is not able to feed herself with utensils. Rapport was established and maintained. Pointing, enlarged materials, and double checking were used to ascertain skill development.

Peabody Picture Vocabulary Test

This instrument is a measure of hearing vocabulary. The child is asked to point to one of four pictures that defines or best describes the word given orally by the examiner. The test pictures were enlarged black and white copies of the test booklet. With Teresa's vision and fine motor coordination factors taken into account, she scored a mental age of 3–2. This is at best only a minimum estimate of her ability due to noted physical factors influencing the evaluation. Teresa knew such words as: pouring, nest, envelope, and goggles. She missed words such as: eagle, tumble, and signal.

Vulpe Assessment Battery

This instrument is a measure of developmental maturity in various areas from birth to 5 years of age.

Area	Age
Gross Motor	10–11 months
Fine Motor	13–24 months
Expressive Auditory Language	18–60 months
Receptive Auditory Language	48–60 months

Cognitive Processes and Specific Concepts

Object Concepts	48–60 months
Body Concepts	30–60 months
Choir Concepts	48–60 months
Shape Concepts	18–54 months
Size Concepts	42 months
Time Concepts	Approximately 60 months
Amount and Number Concepts	48–60 months
Attention and Goal Orientation	48–60 months

Overall, considerable scatter and skill development were evident with Teresa and there were clear indications that she was in the upper ranges of the instrument in a number of areas of cognitive functioning. Skill development was hindered in many areas due to physical factors.

Koontz Child Development Program

This instrument is a measure of developmental maturity from birth to 4 years of age.

Area	Age
Gross Motor	10–12 months
Fine Motor	Approximately 30 months
Social	48 months
Receptive Language	Over 48 months
Expressive Language	42 months

Battelle Developmental Inventory

The Battelle is a standardized, individually administered assessment battery of key developmental skills in children from birth to 8 years. The Cognitive Domain consists of Perceptual Discrimination, Memory, Reasoning and Academic Skills, and Conceptual Development. Perceptual Discrimination and Conceptual Development were administered to Teresa. These sections of the test were the least influenced by Teresa's physical limitations. She scored at the 51% on the Perceptual Discrimination with a DQ of 100. On the Conceptual Development section, she scored at the 9% which yields a DQ of 80. These scores range from the low average to average range.

Adaptive Behavior

On the Vineland Adaptive Behavior Scales, Teresa's scores are heavily influenced by her physical limitations. Her best area of performance was in the receptive language area.

Summary and Recommendations

Based on test results, Teresa's current level of intellectual functioning is in the below average range. She has made such tremendous progress since her last evaluation. Teresa's problems are primarily physical in nature. She has limited gross and fine motor skills and limited oral muscle development for speech. Her hearing as measured by the audiometer indicated normal hearing with a response at each level required for screening. She has a wandering left eye and no one is really sure what she can see and what she can't in the distance. However, Teresa has very good visual perceptual discrimination on the Battelle. Teresa's adaptive behavior is also heavily influenced by her physical limitations, with receptive language her strongest area. Overall test results on the Battelle, Vulpe, and her tremendous progress in school do not support a primary diagnosis of a mental handicap. Teresa is physically disabled with cerebral palsy. Behaviorally, Teresa is stubborn at times, which impedes her progress. An eligibility report for the orthopedically impaired class should be completed.

CASE 3

NAME: Trey Franks
SCHOOL: Home-based
GRADE: Home-based
AGE: 6 weeks old
DOB: 10/28/93
DATE OF EXAMINATION: 12/13/93
Dx: Spina bifida

Summary of Evaluation/Assessment

Patient is performing gross motor activities at approximately a 1-month old level.

STG:

PT: In six months

1. Trey will support weight on forearms. 100%
2. Trey will support weight on hands. 100%
3. Trey will reach for toys on prone hands. 100%
4. Trey will sit independently following positioning for 30 seconds. 100%

LTG:

1. Trey will perform gross motor skills at an 8-month old level.

Rehab Potential: Excellent secondary to parent's involvement in physical therapy program and interest in home exercise program.

Motivation/Attitude: Parent appears very interested in the physical therapy program, mom has degree in special education.

D/C Plans: Discharge will be addressed when long term goals are met.

Physician's changes/comments in treatment plan:

Physician's Signature: _____ Date: _____

Background Information: Patient is being referred by Dr. Croce for physical therapy as needed. Patient was hospitalized for approximately the first three weeks of his life.

Medical Hx: On 10/30/93, patient had removal of myelomeningocele and on 11/6/93 a vp-shunt was placed. Patient required a graft to have closure of myelomeningocele. Patient is now lying on a doughnut to prevent weight bearing along the incision site.

Developmental Hx: Please refer to pediatric case history.

Summary of Clinical/Behavioral Observations: Patient was alert although fussy throughout evaluation process. Patient did not make eye contact with therapist nor did he focus on toys today. Mom states that he is a happy baby and is easy to care for.

Passive Range of Motion: For bilateral upper extremities and lower extremities, is within normal limit. Tightness noted in dorsiflexors.

Muscle Tone: Appears normal in upper extremity, paralysis is noted in bilateral lower extremities and lower trunk.

Gross Motor Milestones: Patient is functioning approximately at 1-month old level demonstrating head bobbing while held at therapist shoulder with slight head righting reactions noted. While in prone position patient is able to rotate head to the left and the right extending enough to clear face. While in supine position patient has difficulty maintaining midline position with head. He is able to turn head to the left and to the right. Patient does not bring hands to midline consistently, nor does he focus on toys or track toys. Head lag present.

Reflexive Reactions: Beginning head control noted while on therapist shoulder. Patient does not demonstrate trunk reactions while prone or supine. ATNR reflex noted to the left when supine.

Recommendation: Home exercise program to include the following:

1. PROM—shoulder adduction, hip adduction
2. Upper extremity weight bearing over roll-towel
3. Head reaction at shoulder
4. Tilting reactions in head while sitting
5. Pull to sit, tucking chin
6. Rolling

INDEX